RADIOLOGY
STRATEGIES

RANJIT BALSÉ, MD

DECEMBER, 2014

RADIOLOGY STRATEGIES

Edited by

Julia R. Fielding

Chief of Abdominal Imaging
Department of Radiology
University of North Carolina
Chapel Hill, North Carolina

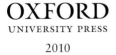

OXFORD
UNIVERSITY PRESS

2010

OXFORD
UNIVERSITY PRESS

Oxford University Press, Inc. publishes works that further
Oxford University's objective of excellence
in research, scholarship and education.

Oxford New York
Auckland Cape Town Dar es Salaam Hong Kong Karachi
Kuala Lumpur Madrid Melbourne Mexico City Nairobi
New Delhi Shanghai Taipei Toronto

With offices in
Argentina Austria Brazil Chile Czech Republic France Greece
Guatemala Hungary Italy Japan Poland Portugal Singapore
South Korea Switzerland Thailand Turkey Ukraine Vietnam

Published by Oxford University Press Inc.
198 Madison Avenue, New York, New York 10016
www.oup.com

Oxford is a registered trade mark of Oxford University Press

Library of Congress Cataloging-in-Publication Data

Radiology strategies / edited by Julia R. Fielding.
p. ; cm.
Includes bibliographical references and index.
ISBN 978-0-19-537119-2 (pbk. : alk. paper)   1. Radiography, Medical.
I. Fielding, Julia R.
   [DNLM: 1. Diagnostic Imaging—methods.   2. Technology,
Radiologic—methods.   WN 180 R128896 2009]
   RC78.R26 2009
   616.07'572—dc22   2009007213

9 8 7 6 5 4 3 2 1

Typeset by Newgen
Printed in China
on acid-free paper

CONTENTS

5 DISEASES OF THE GASTROINTESTINAL TRACT   87
Julia R. Fielding and Wui K. Chong

6 DISEASES OF THE GENITOURINARY TRACT   117
Julia R. Fielding, Wui K. Chong, and Ellie R. Lee

7 DISEASES OF THE MUSCULOSKELETAL SYSTEM   151
NancyM. Major and Taymon Domzalski

8 DISEASES OF THE CARDIOVASCULAR SYSTEM   177
W. Brian Hyslop and Robert Dixon

9 IMAGING OF PEDIATRIC PATIENTS   211
Sarah D. Bixby and Carlo Buonomo

10 A PRIMER ON THE USE OF NUCLEAR MEDICINE TESTS 249

Amir H. Khandani

PREFACE

I have spent the majority of my professional career teaching radiologists—those in practice and those in training. It is one of the greatest joys in academic medicine and one of the most important parts of my career. As imaging becomes more central to diagnosis, more complex, and very expensive it has become increasingly important for a physician to order the correct test to answer a specific clinical question. This book is an attempt to extend pertinent radiology knowledge to our colleagues—the internists, surgeons, family practitioners, and pediatricians who are often on the front line of medical care. My hope is that this book may be of help to them in treating their patients correctly and effectively.

Dr. Julia R. Fielding
February 6, 2009

CONTRIBUTORS

Sarah D. Bixby, MD
Department of Radiology
Children's Hospital
Boston, Massachusetts

Carlo Buonomo, MD
Department of Radiology
Children's Hospital
Boston, Massachusetts

Wui K. Chong, MD, FRCR
Department of Radiology
University of North Carolina
School of Medicine
Chapel Hill, North Carolina

Aamer R. Chughtai, MD
Department of Radiology
Ann Arbor, Michigan

Robert G. Dixon, MD
Department of Radiology
University of North Carolina School
of Medicine
Chapel Hill, North Carolina

Taymon Domzalski, MD
Duke University Medical Center
Durham, North Carolina

Julia R. Fielding, MD
Department of Radiology
University of North Carolina
School of Medicine
Chapel Hill, North Carolina

W. Brian Hyslop, MD, PHD
Department of Radiology
University of North Carolina
School of Medicine
Chapel Hill, North Carolina

Valerie Jewells, DO
Department of Radiology
University of North Carolina
School of Medicine
Chapel Hill, North Carolina

Amir H. Khandani, MD
Associate Professor of Radiology
Director, Nuclear Medicine Residency/Fellowship
Director, PET Services
University of North Carolina
School of Medicine

Ellie Lee, MD
Department of Radiology
University of North Carolina
School of Medicine
Chapel Hill, North Carolina

Nancy M. Major, MD
Department of Radiology
Duke University Medical Center
Durham, North Carolina

Wittaya Padungchaichote, MD
Lopburi Cancer Center
Lopburi, Thailand

Bonnie Yankaskas, PHD
Department of Radiology
University of North Carolina
School of Medicine
Chapel Hill, North Carolina

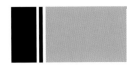

ACKNOWLEDGMENT

The editor acknowledges the invaluable secretarial help of Ms. Virginia Butler.

HOW TO USE THIS BOOK

This book is designed to help health-care providers choose the radiologic test most likely to answer a clinical question. Obviously, no test can replace a careful patient interview and physical examination but radiologic tests have become critical adjuncts for accurate diagnosis of many diseases. For this book, contributing radiologists, all experts in their fields, were asked to choose the most common questions asked of them by their clinical colleagues and recommend the most useful radiologic test or tests.

Clinical chapters are devoted to a specific organ system. Each is composed of 10 clinical vignettes. Because of their unique attributes, nuclear medicine tests and pediatric diagnosis are discussed in separate chapters.

This book can be used in two ways. For specific clinical complaints check the index for a heading such as headache or claudication. The appropriate vignette will give the rationale for and recommend a radiologic test. Two images will be included that demonstrate the abnormality. For some common general complaints, you can review each chapter or refer to the test algorithms.

A caveat, the recommendations in this book are based on expert opinion gleaned from years of practice and review of published data. They are guidelines only, and the referring physician must ultimately choose the best course of action for diagnosis of each patient.

IMAGING ALGORITHMS FOR COMMON CLINICAL PRESENTATIONS

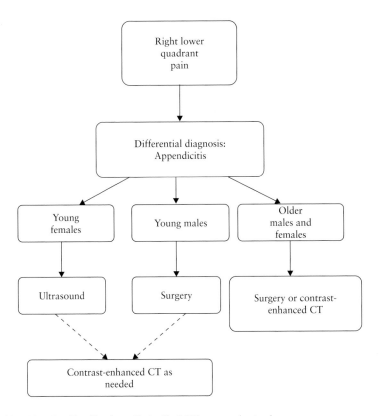

Algorithm 1 Algorithm for patient with right lower quadrant pain.
CT, computed tomography.

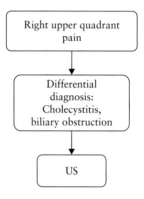

Algorithm 2 Algorithm for patient with right upper quadrant pain.
US, ultrasound.

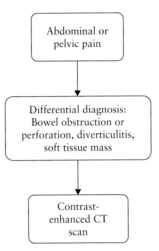

Algorithm 3 Algorithm for patient with abdominal or pelvic pain.
CT, computed tomography.

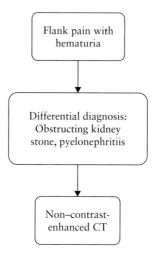

Algorithm 4   Algorithm for patient with flank pain with hematuria.
CT, computed tomography.

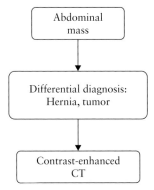

Algorithm 5 Algorithm for patient with abdominal mass.
CT, computed tomography.

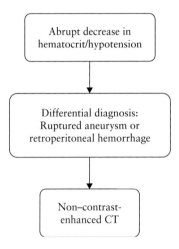

Algorithm 6 Algorithm for patient with abrupt decrease in hematocrit/hypotension. CT, computed tomography.

```
┌─────────────────────┐
│                     │
│       Trauma        │
│                     │
└──────────┬──────────┘
           │
           ▼
╭─────────────────────────╮
│ Contrast-enhanced CT scan of │
│   involved areas with sagittal │
│  reformatted images of bones │
╰─────────────────────────╯
```

Algorithm 7 Algorithm for patient with trauma.
CT, computed tomography.

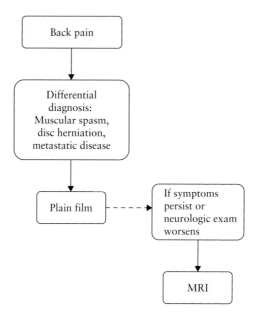

Algorithm 8 Algorithm for patient with back pain. MRI, magnetic resonance imaging.

```
┌─────────────────────────────┐
│     Vaginal bleeding–        │
│   pregnancy test positive    │
└─────────────────────────────┘
              │
              ▼
┌─────────────────────────────┐
│    Differential diagnosis:   │
│     Ectopic pregnancy,       │
│  spontaneous abortion, post- │
│     partum abnormalities     │
└─────────────────────────────┘
              │
              ▼
┌─────────────────────────────┐
│        Transvaginal          │
│            US                │
└─────────────────────────────┘
```

Algorithm 9 Algorithm for female patient with vaginal bleeding and a positive pregnancy test.
US, ultrasound.

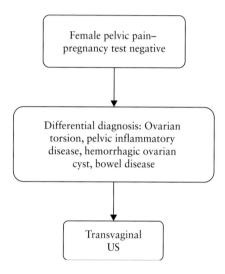

Algorithm 10 Algorithm for female patient with pelvic pain and a negative pregnancy test.
US, ultrasound.

Algorithm 11   Algorithm for cancer staging.
CT, computed tomography; MRI, magnetic resonance imagimg; PET, photon emission tomography.

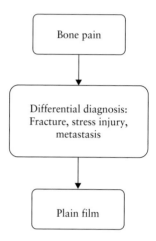

Algorithm 12 Algorithm for patient with bone pain.

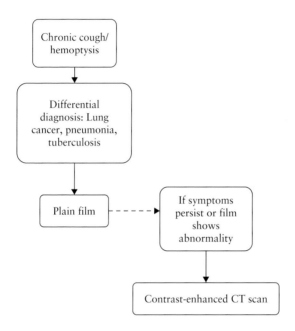

Algorithm 13 Algorithm for patient with chronic cough/hemoptysis. CT, computed tomography.

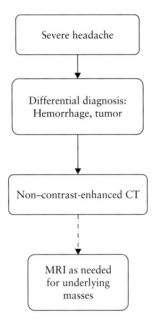

Algorithm 14 Algorithm for patient with severe headache.
CT, computed tomography; MRI, magnetic resonance imaging.

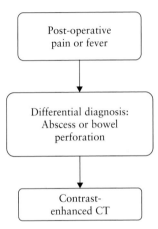

Algorithm 15 Algorithm for patient with post-operative pain or fever.
CT, computed tomography.

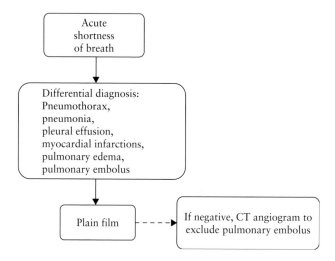

Algorithm 16   Algorithm for patient with acute shortness of breath. CT, computed tomography.

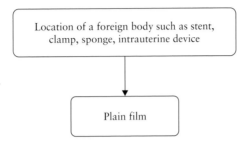

Algorithm 17 Algorithm to determine location of foreign body.

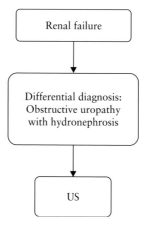

Algorithm 18   Algorithm for patient with renal failure.
US, ultrasound.

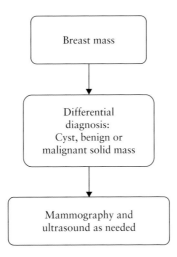

Algorithm 19 Algorithm for patient with breast mass.

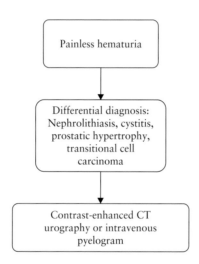

Algorithm 20   Algorithm for patient with painless hematuria. CT, computed tomography.

1

USE OF INTRAVENOUS RADIOGRAPHIC CONTRAST AGENTS

Julia R. Fielding

Iodine-Based Agents

Radiographic contrast agents were developed to increase differences in the absorption rate of x-rays in soft tissues. All available agents consist of a modification of a tri-iodinated benzene ring. Additional components of contrast agents allow large volumes of contrast to be administered quickly and with minimal toxicity. The majority of hospitals use low osmolar contrast agents to decrease osmolality, which is associated with adverse reactions.

NONIONIC MONOMER

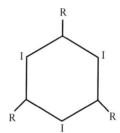

R, hydrophilic, nonionizing side chains; I, Iodine.

USAGE

Iodine-based contrast agents are used for the majority of computed tomography scans and for some fluoroscopic studies, such as the intravenous urogram. They increase the conspicuity of tumors and allow for performance of angiography. The volume injected depends on the scan and ranges from 50 ml to 150 ml. Injectable agents are often administered with oral contrast agents that coat the intestines.

TOXICITY AND PROPHYLAXIS

Adverse reactions to the injection of iodine-based contrast agents occur in approximately 5% of patients and include nausea, vomiting, pruritis, vasovagal episodes, nephrotoxicity, laryngeal edema, and anaphylactic shock. The majority of reactions occur within 15 minutes of administration of the agent. Severe reactions occur in 0.05% of cases and the death rate is 1 case per 75,000 injections. This is similar to the risk profile of penicillin.

In high-risk patients, those with a history of a severe-adverse contrast reaction, active asthma or multiple drug or environmental allergies, the risk of an adverse reaction to a repeat administration of intravenous contrast agent is approximately 15%, or three times baseline. If the examination must be performed, premedication with steroids is recommended to decrease the risk of a second adverse reaction. The current recommendation is 50 mg prednisone PO, 12 and 2 hours before the procedure.

Nephrotoxicity is a significant risk in those patients with insulin-dependent diabetes mellitus and a serum creatinine >1.5 mg/dl. It is prudent to avoid contrast-enhanced studies in these patients. Vigorous intravenous hydration before and after the procedure limits toxicity.

Gadolinium-Based Contrast Agents

These agents were designed to produce the same effects as iodine-based contrast agents, specifically, conspicuity of tumors and vessels. Gadolinium, a rare earth metal, is a toxic agent. It is only when firmly attached to a chelate that it becomes safe to administer intravenously.

USAGE

Gadolinium chelates are administered for virtually all examinations of the brain and soft tissues. They are usually not required for studies of the bones and joints. The volume administered is much less than that for iodine-based agents and is based on weight in kilograms and rarely exceeds 15 ml. At present, oral contrast agents are not usually administered, although Barium and milk can be used.

TOXICITY AND PROPHYLAXIS

The risk of an adverse reaction in a patient with normal renal function is virtually nil. Occasional episodes of vomiting and hives occur, but there have been very few reported cases of anaphylaxis.

In the patient with renal failure, specifically those with serum Cr >3.0 mg/dl and glomerular filtration rate less than 30 ml/min, nephrogenic systemic fibrosis may develop. This disease, first described in 2000, is manifested by skin thickening, joint contractures, and severe pain and may be fatal. Over 200 cases have been reported worldwide. All have been associated with intravenous administration of a gadolinium chelate within 2 or 3 months before onset of symptoms. The risk of contracting the disease increased with repeat examinations. The use of gadolinium chelates is to be avoided whenever possible in patients with moderate to severe renal failure.

BIBLIOGRAPHY

Kanal E, Barkvich AJ, Bell C, et al. ACR Guidance document for safe MR practices: 2007. *AJR*. 2007;188:1447-1474.

Lasser E, Berry C, Talner L, et al. Pretreatment with corticosteroids to alleviate reactions to intravenous contrast material. *NEJM*. 1987; 317:845-849.

2

VALUE OF DIAGNOSTIC TESTS

Bonnie Yankaskas

You see a 50-year-old woman with a negative family history of breast cancer. You recommend that she have screening mammography. You get the report and she has had a positive mammogram and the radiologist recommends that she return for further imaging. The report says that calcifications were seen and to determine appropriate follow-up, further imaging is recommended. From the literature you know that in a 50-year-old woman, with negative family history of breast cancer, the positive predictive value of a positive mammogram is approximately 3%–5%.

What does the positive predictive value tell you?

1. that if she has cancer, there is a 3%–5% chance it will be detected
2. that she has a 3%–5% risk of breast cancer in the next year
3. that there is a 3%–5% probability that a positive mammogram implies presence of cancer
4. that there is a 3%–5% probability that the positive mammogram was incorrect (no cancer present)

The answer is 3.

If the woman was 70 years old what would the positive predictive value be in comparison to the 3%–5%?

1. higher
2. lower
3. the same
4. cannot tell

The correct answer is 1. Predictive values are affected by prevalence of disease. Older women have a higher prevalence of disease than younger women, and the predictive value is higher. Thus a positive mammogram in an older woman has a higher probability of predicting presence of cancer.

The accuracy measures used for diagnostic testing include the following:

Sensitivity—the probability of a positive mammogram assessment, when cancer is present.
Specificity—the probability of a negative mammogram assessment, when cancer is absent.
Positive predictive value (PPV)—the probability of cancer when the mammographic assessment is positive.
Negative predictive value (NPV)—the probability of no cancer when the mammographic assessment is negative.

To calculate these measures, we usually create a 2 × 2 table as shown in the following Table 2.1:

Table 2.1 Example of a 2 × 2 Table

	Cancer present	Cancer absent
Mammogram +	TP	FP
Mammogram −	FN	TN

FN, false negative; FP, false positive; TN, true negative; TP, true positive.

True positive (TP) means the mammogram was positive and there was cancer.

False negative (FN) means the mammogram was negative and there was cancer.

False positive (FP) means the mammogram was positive and there was no cancer.

True negative (TN) means the mammogram was negative and there was no cancer.

Sensitivity is based on the denominator of all cancer and is calculated as TP/TP + FN.

Specificity is based on the denominator of all non-cancer and is calculated as TN/TN + FP.

Sensitivity and specificity are considered characteristics of the test, and should be stable across the population.

PPV is based on the denominator of all positive test results and is calculated as TP/TP + FP.

NPV is based on the denominator of all negative test results and is calculated as TN/TN + FN.

Predictive value will be affected by prevalence of disease (all disease/total tests). Prevalence of disease (or cancer in this case) is the proportion of the population tested that has the disease (TP + FN)/(TP + FN + FP + TN). As prevalence increases, the PPV will increase and the NPV decrease. An example follows in Tables 2.2 and 2.3.

Choose your test based on its sensitivity and specificity. With sensitivity and specificity constant, differences in the prevalence of disease in a tested

Table 2.2 PPV when Prevalence of Cancer Is 5 per 1,000

	Cancer present	Cancer absent	
Mammogram +	43	398	441
Mammogram −	7	9,552	9,559
	50	9,950	10,000

FN, false negative; FP, false positive; PPV, positive predictive value; TN, true negative; TP, true positive.
Sens = 85%; Spec = 96%; Prevalence = 5/1,000; PPV = 6.8%

Table 2.3 PPV when Cancer Prevalence Is 10 per 1,000

	Cancer present	Cancer absent	
Mammogram +	85	496	581
Mammogram −	15	9,504	9,519
	100	9,900	10,000

FN, false negative; FP, false positive; PPV, positive predictive value; TN, true negative; TP, true positive.
Sens = 85%; Spec = 96%; Prevalence = 10/1,000; PPV = 14.6%

population will affect the PPV. To rule out a diagnosis, choose a test with high sensitivity to minimize FN results. To rule in a diagnosis choose a test with high specificity to minimize FP results.

3

DISEASES OF THE HEAD, NECK, BRAIN, AND NERVOUS SYSTEM

Valerie Jewells and
Wui K. Chong

3-1. Spinal Tumor

CASE HISTORY

A 74-year-old woman presents with back pain and known history of breast cancer. A magnetic resonance imaging (MRI) of the total spine was performed.

BACKGROUND

Tumors in the spinal region are typically due to metastatic disease to the vertebral bodies. The most common causes of metastases are breast, lung, and prostate cancer, followed by multiple myeloma, lymphoma, and renal cell carcinoma. Metastases can also involve only the leptomeninges or epidural space as frequently occurs with drop metastases from central nervous system (CNS) tumors of the brain such as ependymomas and medulloblastomas, but can even be seen with glioblastoma multiformae. Primary tumors of the spinal cord are much less common than metastatic disease, and are typically of two types: astrocytomas (predominantly cervical and thoracic) and ependymomas (most common at the conus). Spinal cord tumors usually involve multiple segments, and so the differential diagnosis includes transverse myelitis, cord infarct, multiple sclerosis, and cord edema from vascular malformation or dual AV fistula. Primary bone tumors of the spine range from benign aneursymal bone cysts and osteoid osteomas to rare malignant chordomas, sacral teratomas, and sarcomas.

TEST RATIONALE

Metastatic and primary tumors of the spine are best evaluated with MRI because of superior visualization of the extent of vertebral body, paraspinal muscle, and meningeal/epidural tumor, thus adequately assessing the degree of spinal canal and neural foraminal stenosis and guiding surgical intervention and radiation therapy. Most metastases on MRI will be low signal on T1 and bright on T2 and enhance postcontrast injection (see Fig. 3-1A). Computed tomography (CT) with myelography can be used in patients for whom MRI cannot be performed, that is, morbidly obese patients who cannot fit in the magnet, as well as patients with claustrophobia or cardiac pacemakers. CT, however, will consistently underestimate disease extent compared to MRI. A spinal cord tumor is depicted (see Fig. 3-1B) which would be very difficult to visualize with CT.

TEST OF CHOICE

Contrast-enhanced MRI.

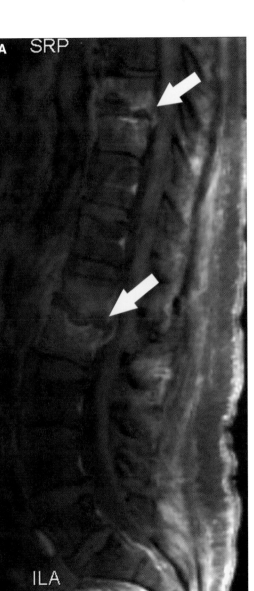

Figure 3-1A   A sagittal T1 post contrast image of the lumbar spine demonstrates metastatic enhancing lesions to the T9, T10, L1, and L2 vertebral bodies. There is minimal extension into the epidural space as tumor breaks through the posterior vertebral body cortex (see arrows). Note that there is disc space preservation and lack of disc involvement, typical for tumor, but not typical for discitis.

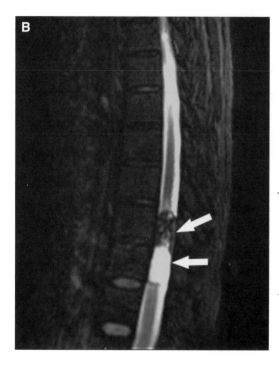

Figure 3-1B   A sagittal T2 image of the lower thoracic spine in a different patient, a 25-year-old male reveals a primary spinal cord tumor. This image demonstrates a mixed solid (upper arrow) and cystic (lower arrow) lesion of the thoracic cord. The very dark signal of the solid portion suggests hemosiderin from previous hemorrhage. There can also be an associated syrinx with spinal cord tumors, not seen in this case.

BIBLIOGRAPHY

Smith JK, Lury K, Castillo M. Imaging of spinal and spinal cord tumors. *Semin Roentgenol.* 2006;41(4):274-293.

Andreula C, Murrone M. Metastatic disease of the spine. *Eur Radiol.* 2005 Mar;15(3):627-632. Epub 2005 Feb 5. Review.

3-2. Brain Tumor

CASE HISTORY
A 22-year-old male patient presents with new-onset seizure.

BACKGROUND
Brain tumors are divided into pediatric tumors, which predominantly involve the posterior fossa, and adult tumors, which predominantly involve the supratentorial regions. Adult malignant tumors are most commonly derived from glial cell lines, and therefore three types are most commonly seen—astrocytomas, oligodendrogliomas (see Figs.3-2A and 3-2B), or the more common and higher-grade glioblastoma multiformae tumors. Since these tumors are of glial origin, they predominantly arise in the white matter of the cerebral hemispheres. Less common neuronal origin tumors in adults include gangliogliomas, ganglioneuromas, and gangliocytomas, which all involve the gray matter. A very common benign intracranial tumor in adults is a meningioma, which arises from the meninges, and so remains in contact with the meninges. Less commonly, immunocompromised patients may develop non-Hodgkins lymphoma, which has a tendency to cross the midline into the opposite hemisphere via white matter tracts, and predominently involves the white matter. Metastases are always within the differential when there is a brain mass, particularly when there are multiple masses. Metastases predominantly lie at the gray–white matter junctions, with 80% being found in the cerebral hemispheres, while 10%–15% deposit in the cerebellum, and only 2%–3% are found in the brainstem. Metastases to brain occur with the following frequencies for different primary tumors: lung, 35%–64%; breast, 14%–18%; melanoma, 4%–21%; renal and colon, 5%–9.5%; and unknown primary, 5%–11%.

TEST RATIONALE
Brain tumors can be followed with CT, but MRI with contrast enhancement is the preferred and more sensitive test. Both perfusion MRI and MR spectroscopy (MRS) are newer methods of assessment of brain tumors. When using MRS, metastatic lesions demonstrate a well-defined spectroscopic abnormality compared to the infiltrative nature seen in primary brain tumors. Typical metabolic abnormalities seen with MRS in brain tumors include reductions in N-acetyl-aspartate (NAA) due to loss of neurons, elevated lipid and lactate portending a more aggressive tumor/necrosis, and choline indicating rapid cell turnover. Measurement of these metabolites also assists in the evaluation of patients posttherapy for areas of recurrence.

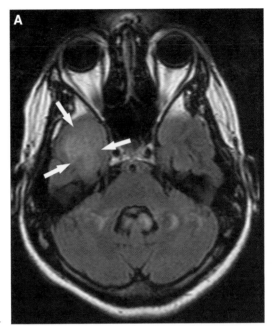

Figures 3-2A and 3-2B The fluid attenuation inversion recovery (FLAIR) image reveals an increased signal poorly defined mass involving the right temporal lobe with sulcal effacement from edema (arrows define the margins). Likewise, the postcontrast image demonstrates subtle peripheral enhancement. The location of the tumor and age of the patient are not uncommon for a ganglioglioma or gangliocytoma, which often present with seizures. However, there is extensive white matter involvement, which is atypical for these diagnoses. Oligodenrogliomas not uncommonly involve the gray and white matter, and was the diagnosis in this case.

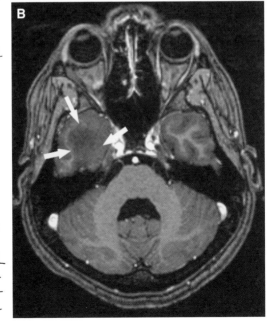

MR perfusion can also assist in the diagnosis of tumors and help with differentiation of recurrence from radiation therapy changes. Evaluation of the cerebral blood flow maps typically demonstrates hyperperfusion in areas of tumor recurrence, and hypoperfusion in areas of radiation necrosis.

TEST OF CHOICE
Contrast-enhanced MRI.

BIBLIOGRAPHY
Poussaint TY. Magnetic resonance imaging of pediatric brain tumors: state of the art. *Top Magn Reson Imaging.* 2001 Dec;12(6):411-433. Review.

Sugahara T, Korogi Y, Tomiguchi S, et al. Posttherapeutic intraaxial brain tumor: the value of perfusion-sensitive contrast-enhanced MR imaging for differentiating tumor recurrence from nonneoplastic contrast-enhancing tissue. *AJNR Am J Neuroradiol.* 2000 May;21(5):901-909.

3-3. Intracranial Infections

CASE HISTORY

A 34-year-old patient presents to the emergency room (ER) with fever and changes in mental status. A CT was performed that yielded insufficient information, and subsequently an MRI with contrast was obtained.

BACKGROUND

There are multiple types of intracranial infections, including meningitis, encephalitis, brain abscess, and ventriculitis/ependymitis. These are secondary to infection of the meninges, brain, and ventricular ependymal lining respectively. Intracranial infection can arise from contiguous or hematogenous spread. Contiguous spread is usually from the adjacent paranasal sinuses (particularly frontal) or the mastoid air cells of the temporal bone, and can result in brain abscess, or in the case of mastoid origin, sigmoid sinus thrombosis and brain infarction. Bacterial meningitis can occur via contiguous or hematogenous spread. The origin of hematogenous brain infection is often cardiac, but can also be pulmonary, renal/bladder, or secondary to osteomyelitis. Hematogenous abscesses usually occur at the gray–white matter junctions as ring-enhancing lesions as a result of the infectious material lodging in peripheral small vessels. Immunocompromised patients are predisposed to brain infections often not seen in other patient groups. Encephalitis due to *Toxoplasmosis gondii* and *Coccidiodes immitis* may also involve the spinal cord/nerve roots and choroid plexus of the lateral ventricle. A common infection with only a 6-month survival rate in patients with human immunovirus (HIV)/acquired immunodeficiency syndrome (AIDS) results in diffuse white matter changes as progressive multifocal leukoencephalopathy (PML). The infectious agent is the JC papovavirus.

TEST RATIONALE

The preferred method of evaluation of central nervous system (CNS) infection is multiplanar MRI with contrast enhancement (see Figs. 3-3A and 3-3B). Although CT can be used, MR is a more sensitive and specific test, particularly for subtle findings. Infections of the brain parenchyma are often ring-enhancing lesions, whereas those of the meninges show thickening and enhancement adjacent to the brain. Dilation of the ventricles, hydrocephalus, is often present. Of note, diffusion imaging also helps narrow the differential diagnosis since abcesses often demonstrate restricted diffusion within the brain. In addition, MR spectroscopy can assist with differentiation of bacterial infections from tuberculosis and fungal causes—specifically, the presence of lipid and lactate in tubercular abcesses; lipid,

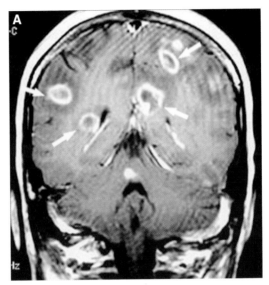

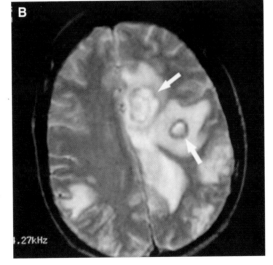

Figures 3-3A and 3-3B
The coronal postcontrast MRI image reveals ring-enhancing lesions (arrows), while the associated surrounding white matter edema is low in signal. Whereas the vasogenic edema from the lesions (arrows) is bright on axial T2 images. A not dissimilar appearance can be seen with septic emboli of which *Staphylococcus aureus* is the most common offending agent. Bacterial infections can, however, also exhibit adjacent daughter nodules, which will help differentiate the cause as infectious not metastatic.

lactate, and amino acids in fungal abcesses; and cytosolic acids, acetate, and succinate in pyogenic abcesses.

TEST OF CHOICE
Contrast-enhanced MRI.

BIBLIOGRAPHY
Offiah CE, Turnbull IW. The imaging appearances of intracranial CNS infections in adult HIV and AIDS patients. *Clin Radiol.* 2006 May;61(5):393-401. Review.
Luthra G, Parihar A, Nath K, et al. Comparative evaluation of fungal, tubercular, and pyogenic brain abscesses with conventional and diffusion MR imaging and proton MR spectroscopy. *AJNR.* 2007 Aug;28(7):1332-1338.

3-4. Head Trauma

CASE HISTORY
A 4-month-old infant is brought to the ER by her mother. The infant was "not acting right after rolling off of the couch onto a carpeted floor."

BACKGROUND
The most common causes of head trauma are motor vehicle accidents, altercations, and falls. Multiple different types of hemorrhage are seen with head trauma. The most common is a subdural hematoma, which demonstrates a concentric convex outward configuration crossing suture lines, and is confined to the extra-axial subdural space. Epidural hematomas occur less commonly than subdural hematomas, and frequently arise from a middle meningeal artery tear. Epidural hematomas do not cross the sutures, are biconvex, and compress the brain away from the hematoma. Unlike epidural and subdural hematomas, subarachnoid hemorrhage is located deep to the meninges and extends into the sulci and cisterns, while traumatic brain contusions are confined to the parenchyma and are commonly seen in the bifrontal/ bitemporal regions and the pons as a result of the brain striking the adjacent calvarum. Diffuse axonal injury most often occurs at gray–white matter parenchymal junctions and within the corpus callosum. This type of injury is secondary to the gray and white matter of the brain decelerating at different rates, resulting in a tearing of small vessels and axons at the junction. The small resultant hemorrhages best seen with susceptibility weighted or T2* images. Concussion and postconcussion syndromes demonstrate no CT or conventional MRI findings.

TEST RATIONALE
Imaging in head trauma is typically performed with noncontrasted CT in the ER. The density of hemorrhage changes with time. Initially bright on CT, blood becomes isodense at approximately 3 days to 1 week postinjury, and then low density by several months postinjury (see Figs. 3-4A and 3-4B). MRI may be of assistance in complex cases or for visualization of subtle hemorrhages.

TEST OF CHOICE
Non–contrast-enhanced CT scan.

BIBLIOGRAPHY
Davis P. Expert panel on neurologic imaging. Head trauma. *AJNR*. 2007 Sep;28(8):1619-1621. Review.
Gallagher CN, Hutchinson PJ, Pickard JD. Neuroimaging in trauma. *Curr Opin Neurol*. 2007 Aug;20(4):403-409. Review.

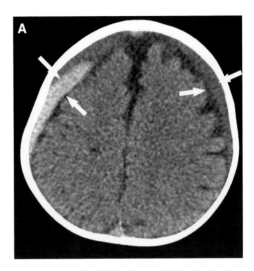

Figure 3-4A   The arrows are marking bilateral crescent-shaped collections of blood in the extra-axial spaces, specifically the subdural space. The collection on the right has bright acute blood superimposed upon blood that is subacute in nature. The left-sided subdural is subacute since its attenuation is almost equal to that of the underlying brain. Owing to the fact that the subdural blood is both acute and subacute, more than one incidence of trauma is suspected, and the patient and her family were referred to social services for possible child abuse.

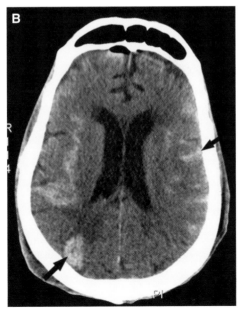

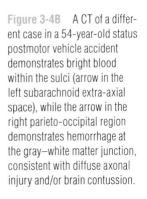

Figure 3-4B   A CT of a different case in a 54-year-old status postmotor vehicle accident demonstrates bright blood within the sulci (arrow in the left subarachnoid extra-axial space), while the arrow in the right parieto-occipital region demonstrates hemorrhage at the gray–white matter junction, consistent with diffuse axonal injury and/or brain contussion.

3-5. Head and Neck Imaging

CASE HISTORY
A 55-year-old male presents to his family physician with a left-sided neck mass. His physician orders a CT with contrast for further evaluation.

BACKGROUND
There are many types of masses that arise in the neck, but most commonly, these masses are related to malignancy. The most common type of head and neck cancer is squamous cell carcinoma (SCCA) arising from the mucosal surfaces of the nasopharynx (NP), nasal cavity, paranasal sinuses, oropharynx, hypopharynx, and supraglottic, glottic, or infraglottic regions. Many of these patients present with painless metastases to lymph nodes (see Fig. 3-5A). These cancers are predominantly seen in smokers and those who abuse alcohol, but, in the case of nasopharyngeal tumors, can be secondary to human papilloma virus infection. Less common sites of head and neck cancer include salivary/lacrimal gland tumors of varying pathologies and prognosis including pleomorphic adenoma (benign but locally aggressive), adenoid cystic and mucoepidermoid cancer (malignant), or less commonly Warthin's tumor (benign). Lymphoma often presents with neck masses from lymphadenopathy. Pre- and postseptal orbital cellulits and facial cellulitis from dental or sinus infections are not uncommon causes of swelling/masses in children and adults. An uncommon neck mass is a carotid body tumor, which occurs at the carotid bifurcation and is a neuroendocrine paraganglioma similar to tumors of the same pathology seen in the adrenal and para-aortic abdominal regions (see Fig. 3-5B).

TEST RATIONALE
All head and neck pathologies can be readily evaluated with contrast-enhanced CT. Imaging is needed to stage these malignancies because complete extent and nodal metastases may not be evident to the clinician. It is best for CT images to be obtained in both bone and soft tissue windows, and acquired in the axial plane with coronal and sagittal reformatted images. Tumors of the NP region, salivary glands, and skin cancers suspected of perineural or intracranial spread are however best imaged with contrast-enhanced MRI in three planes to assess the course of cranial nerves V and VII. In addition, photon emission tomography-computed tomography (PET-CT) is a useful tool for imaging head and neck cancers. It is particularly useful for cases of unknown primary, second primary, and unsuspected metastases.

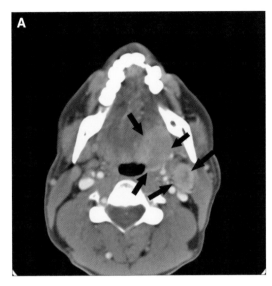

Figure 3-5A   This CT of the patient in the aforementioned case report demonstrates a
left tongue base and root of tongue cancer with anterior tonsilar pillar involvement (anterior
three arrows encircle the mass) and a ring-enhancing metastatic lesion at level IIA on the
left (two posterior arrows) in the paraphyngeal space. The IIA adenopathy was the palpable
mass resulting in the patient's presentation. This metastatic lymph node demonstrates
necrosis, and likely has perilymphatic spread because of its poorly defined margins.
Lymphadenopathy reduces the patient's prognosis to a 50% 5-year survival while extra-
nodal spread reduces the prognosis even further to 25%.

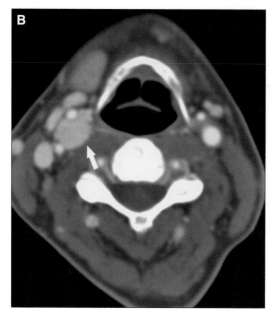

Figure 3-5B This image depicts a right-sided carotid body tumor or paraganglioma seen in another patient presenting with a neck mass. The tumor splays the contrast-enhancing internal (anterior) and external (posterior) branches of the carotid artery. These tumors enhance avidly, commonly equal to the adjacent vessels owing to their significant blood supply from the ascending pharyngeal artery.

TEST OF CHOICE
Contrast-enhanced CT scan.

BIBLIOGRAPHY
Gor DM, Langer JE, Loevner LA. Imaging of cervical lymph nodes in head and neck cancer: the basics. *Radiol Clin North Am.* 2006 Jan;44(1): 101-110, viii. Review.
Corry J, Rischin D, Hicks RJ, et al. The role of PET-CT in the management of patients with advanced cancer of the head and neck. *Curr Oncol Rep.* 2008 Mar;10(2):149-155.

3-6. Stroke

CASE HISTORY

A 35-year-old male patient presents to the ER with new-onset stumbling and vertigo 12 hours after falling from a ladder.

BACKGROUND

There are two major types of strokes—embolic and hemorrhagic. Most strokes are embolic and are due to occlusion of a cerebral vessel by a clot originating from plaque in the carotid artery or aorta. Less commonly, embolic strokes arise as a result of carotid or vertebral dissection. Hemorrhagic strokes are often secondary to hypertension. Rather uncommon causes of stroke include hypoperfusion/hypoxic encephalopathy, venous infarction, amyloid angiopathy (occur in the elderly, and often have associated hemorrhage), vasculitis, fibromuscular dysplasia, and posterior reversible encephalopathy syndrome (PRES). The window of opportunity for treating an embolic stroke is 1–6 hours for intravenous thrombolytic therapy, and 1–4 hours for catheter-directed thrombolysis and/or clot retrieval. Without therapy, dismal outcomes are the rule, including death in 10%–15%, long-term disability in 30%–50%, and institutionalization in 20%–25%. Thrombolytic therapy can only be administered if the area of stroke involves less than one-third the territory of the middle cerebral artery, no mass effect is present, and there is no evidence of hemorrhage on CT.

TEST RATIONALE

Imaging of stroke can be performed with both CT and MRI. CT is typically used in the acute setting to determine stroke extent and presence or absence of hemorrhage. Early findings on CT scan range from a normal examination to a hyperdense artery, insular/cortical blurring, disappearing lentiform nucleus, or most commonly hypoattenuation in the region of infarct. CT angiography can also demonstrate an intraarterial clot, and CT perfusion can delineate the area of abnormal perfusion. MRI demonstrates restricted diffusion at 1 hour following the embolic event, and often reveals small lacunar infarcts not seen with CT (see Fig.3-6A). Abnormal T2 bright signal will also be seen by 2–3 hours postinfarct on MRI, and low T1 signal (see Fig.3-6B) as well as possible meningeal enhancement is often identified by 24 hours. Perfusion MRI can demonstrate the area of hypoperfusion, which can be larger, or "mismatch" the diffusion abnormality, demonstrating that there is an area of brain at risk, that is, an

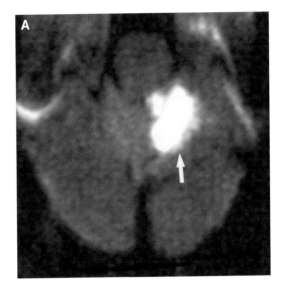

Figure 3-6A   Diffusion imaging demonstrating very bright signal in the region of infarct (arrow) that had a matching low area of signal on the apparent diffusion coefficient (ADC) map consistent with restricted diffusion and acute to sub-acute infarct.

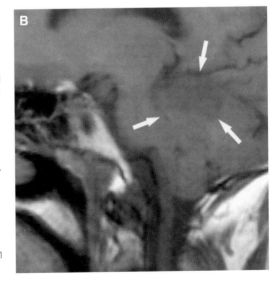

Figure 3-6B   Sagittal T1 image revealing an area of low signal in the superior left cerebellum (arrow) from a superior cerebellar artery infarction and resultant cytotoxic edema. There were matching bright T2 abnormalities in this region. MRA of the neck performed at the same imaging session demonstrated a dissection of the left vertebral artery.

"ischemic penumbra" that has not yet infarcted, and can possibly be saved with appropriate intervention. Perfusion abnormalities can also be seen in areas at risk before the infarct occurs because of vascular insufficiency from atherosclerotic disease.

TEST OF CHOICE
CT scan with and without contrast.

BIBLIOGRAPHY
Neuann-Haefelin T, Steinmetz H. Time is brain: is MRI the clock? *Curr Opin Neurol.* 2007 Aug;20(4):410-416. Review.

Camargo EC, Furie KL, Singhal AB, et al. Acute brain infarct: detection and delineation with CT angiographic source images versus nonenhanced CT scans. *Radiology.* 2007 Aug;244(2):541-548. Epub 2007 Jun 2.

3-7. Spinal Trauma

CASE HISTORY

An 18-year-old unrestrained male driver presented to the ER with lower extremity weakness after striking a tree and being ejected from the car. The plain films of the thoracic spine revealed anterior displacement of T10 on T11. MRI was performed.

BACKGROUND

Currently, the majority of patients who present to our ER receive a complete CT of the spine if unconscious, or if neurologic symptoms exist. These spinal CT scans are usually reconstructed from a CT of the chest, abdomen, and pelvis obtained to assess organ injury. Younger patients particularly those >10 years of age are predisposed to ligamentous and cord injury without the presence of fracture. Pediatric patients therefore require MRI if symptoms are not explained by radiographic or CT findings. MRI is less sensitive than CT for identification of fracture but is excellent for assessment of disc, ligament, and cord injury. It is particularly important to identify cord transection, displacement, and hematoma quickly so that appropriate treatment can be initiated (see Figs. 3-7A and 3-7B).

TEST OF CHOICE

CT followed by MRI as clinically indicated.

BIBLIOGRAPHY

Antevil JL, Sise MJ, Sack DI, et al. Spiral computed tomography for the initial evaluation of spine trauma: A new standard of care? *J Trauma.* 2006 Aug;61(2):382-387.

Goradia D, Linnau KF, Cohen WA, et al. Correlation of MR imaging findings with intraoperative findings after cervical spine trauma. *AJNR Am J Neuroradiol.* 2007 Feb;28(2):209-215.

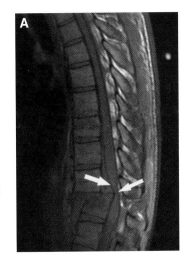

Figure 3-7A Sagittal T1 image of the lower thoracic spine; reveals anterior displacement of T10 on T11, resulting in impingement upon the thoracic cord (arrows) and cord edema. There is also significant edema involving the T11 vertebral body and an anterior corner fracture of T11. There is no bright signal within the spinal cord to suggest hemorrhage.

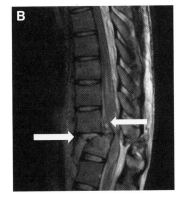

Figure 3-7B T2 sagittal image of the lower thoracic spine; demonstrates complete disruption of the anterior longitudinal ligament (ALL) (anterior arrow), and posterior longitudinal ligament (PLL) (posterior arrow), consistent with three column injury due to a fracture-dislocation. In addition, there is near complete transection of the spinal cord with associated increased T2 signal from cord edema.

3-8. Spinal Discogenic Disease

CASE HISTORY
A 32-year-old patient presents with sudden onset of left lower extremity weakness and low back pain after falling on the ice.

BACKGROUND
The intervertebral discs are commonly affected by many disease processes, ranging from degenerative changes to annular tear, disc bulge, disc herniation, inflammatory end plate changes, and even infection of the disc (discitis). The majority of disc disease presents as bulges or herniations with the formation of bone spurs called osteophytes. Most patients with back pain are treated conservatively. If back or extremity pain is severe then imaging is performed.

TEST RATIONALE
Intervertebral discs are best identified on MR images. The presence of a change in the disc signal to a darker signal on T2 imaging is seen with disc degeneration. This is due to loss of water in the disc. If the degeneration results in a tear of the annulus fibrosis (outer layer) of the disc, then bright signal is seen at the disc margin. As the tear increases in size, then a disc herniation occurs (see Figs. 3-8A and 3-8B). If the annulus fibrosis is weak but intact then a broad-based disc bulge will be seen. The presence of abnormal signal in the end plates of the adjacent vertebral bodies is consistent with fatty (bright T1/dark T2), inflammatory (bright T2, variable T1), or calcific (dark T1 & T2) changes in the endplates. These end plate changes can also result in back pain as can adjacent facet arthritis.

TEST OF CHOICE
Non contrast-enhanced MRI.

BIBLIOGRAPHY
Modic MT, Ross JS. Lumbar degenerative disk disease. *Radiology.* 2007 Oct;245(1):43-61. Review.

Rumbolt Z. Degenerative disorders of the spine. *Semin Roentgenol.* 2006;41(4):327-362.

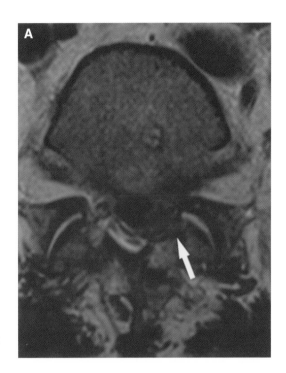

Figure 3-8A Axial T1-weighted MRI demonstrates severe central canal and left lateral recess narrowing from this large herniation (arrow).

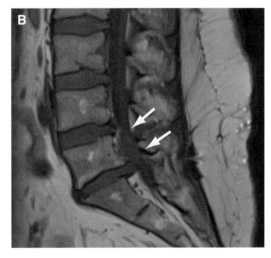

Figure 3-8B A sagittal T1-weighted MRI reveals a large disc herniation at the L5–S1 level with superior migration of disc material (arrows).

3-9. Multiple Sclerosis

CASE HISTORY

A 32-year-old female patient who is wheelchair bound presents to the ER and states that she has new numbness and tingling in her arms.

BACKGROUND

Multiple sclerosis (MS) is an autoimmune disease resulting from diffuse demyelination, axonal transaction/destruction, and neuronal loss. MS is more common in females of northern European extraction, but can be found in all racial and ethnic groups, as well as male patients, who typically present at a later age. The onset of disease is variable, and can be anywhere from the age of 8 into the sixth decade, although most patients present in their 20s–40s. MS is defined as a disease that changes in time and space since recurrent relapsing MS is the most typical form, although progressive nonrelapsing forms also exist. MS can present with any symptom that could be associated with CNS malfunction, but 50% of patients will have optic neuritis as a component of the disease at some time in their life. Neuromyelitis optica is a variant of MS that affects only the optic nerves and spinal cord, although MS proper involves the brain with variable spinal cord and optic nerve involvement. Spinal cord lesions usually result in more obvious clinical symptoms of motor and sensory deficits than brain lesions. The majority of MS patients also have cognitive deficits and usually complain about severe fatigue due to the diffuse nature of this disease. The symptoms may be exacerbated by a flu, stress, or warmer climate.

TEST RATIONALE

Imaging in MS is only to be performed with MRI. Contrasted examinations are preferred, although only approximately 5% of lesions will enhance at any time point, even with an acute attack. The diagnosis of MS is made using clinical findings, assessment of spinal fluid, and MRI changes according to the revised McDonald criteria. A classic MS lesion is bright on T2, globular in configuration, and periventicular in location (see Figs. 3-9A and 3-9B). Lesions often occur in the brain and spinal cord at the same time, so imaging of both regions is often required.

TEST OF CHOICE

Contrast-enhanced MRI.

BIBLIOGRAPHY

McAlpine's Multiple Sclerosis. 4th edition. Philadelphia: Churchill Livingstone Elsevier, 2006.

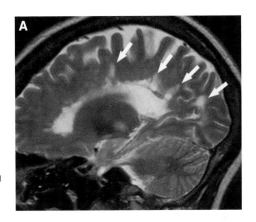

Figure 3-9A A sagittal T2 image at the level of the lateral ventricle demonstrates multiple periventricular lesions (arrows), many globular in configuration, and some with a radiating (Dawson's fingers) appearance. Many other lesions are also seen on this and other images of the brain.

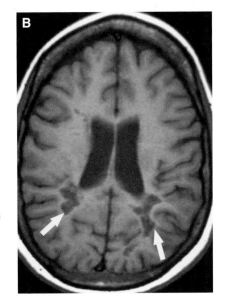

Figure 3-9B An axial T1 image at the level of the lateral ventricles demonstrates biatrial areas of low density consistent with "black holes" (arrows) meaning extensive neuronal loss from burned out MS plaques.

Tortorella P, Rocca MA, Mezzapesa DM, et al. MRI quantification of gray and white matter damage in patients with early-onset multiple sclerosis. *J Neurol.* 2006;253:903-907.

3-10. Congenital Central Nervous System Disease

CASE HISTORY
A 6-month-old female presents with developmental delay.

BACKGROUND
Congenital disease of the CNS is varied in presentation. Early in development, abnormalities of dorsal induction/neurulation can occur within the brain and spinal cord, resulting in adhesions between the ectodermal and endodermal structures. Spinal dorsal induction disorders include closed spinal dysraphism, (tethered cord, tight filum, intradural lipomas, diastematomyelia, and caudal agenesis), as well as open dysraphisms (spina bifida), which include, but are not limited to, lipomeningoceles, lipomyeloceles, meningoceles, and meningomyelocele (see Fig. 3-10A). Chiari II abnormalities in the brain are often associated with these spinal entities. In Chiari II, the cerebellum is displaced inferiorly, the cerebral aqueduct compressed, and hydrocephalus develops. Other induction disorders involving the brain include encephaloceles, nasal gliomas, anencephaly, congenital fissures of the skull and spine, and dermal sinus tracts. Likewise, ventral induction abnormalities such as septoptic dysplasia and holoprosencephaly also occur early in utero, and are often associated with facial abnormalities. Less commonly seen are parenchymal abnormalities of myelination, which usually present several months after birth, are due to genetic abnormalities, and have names like metachromic leukodystrophy, adrenoleukodystrophy (see Fig. 3-10B), and Krabbe's disease. More common extra-axial intracranial abnormalities include arachnoid cysts, epidermoids, dermoids, teratomas, neuroepithelial cysts, Rathke's cleft cysts (sellar/suprasellar region), and lipomas. Finally, aqueductal stenosis with hydrocephalus occurs due to a web, or stenosis, resulting in obstruction of the cerebral aqueduct.

TEST RATIONALE
Suffice it to say that text books are written on this subject, and although many of these developmental anomalies can be seen with CT, they are best imaged with MRI due to improved visualization, and in the interest of preventing unnecessary radiation exposure. None of these entities will require administration of intravenous contrast material for adequate demonstration.

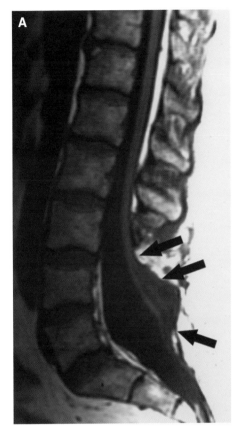

Figure 3-10A   A sagittal T1 image of the lumbar spine demonstrates spinal dysraphism with dilatation of the spinal canal, deficiency of the posterior elements, a low lying conus, and tethering of the distal cord to a posterior neural placode. The skin surface is intact, and therefore, a meningomyelocele is not present.

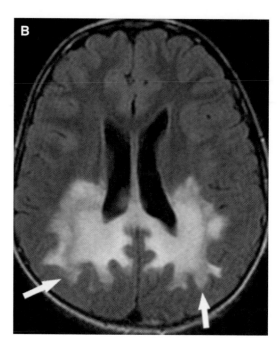

Figure 3-10B   There are bilaterally symmetric areas of increased T2 signal in the peri-artial regions in this 6-month-old patient. This is a rare dysmyelinating disease known as adrenoleukodystrophy.

TEST OF CHOICE
Contrast-enhanced MRI.

BIBLIOGRAPHY
Rossi A, Gandolfo C, Morana G, et al. Current classification and imaging of congenital spinal abnormalities. *Semin Roentgenol.* 2006 Oct;41(4):250-273. Review.
Barkovich AJ. Pediatric Neuroimaging. 2000; Chapter 5; Congenital Malformation of the Brain and Spine:251-381.

3-11. Thyroid Nodule

CASE HISTORY
A 40-year-old female presents with palpable or incidentally discovered thyroid mass.

BACKGROUND
Thyroid nodules are found in approximately 50% of the population. Only 5% of thyroid nodules are palpable; far more are visible with sonography or CT, both of which can detect nodules that are only millimeters in size (see Fig. 3-11). The vast majority of thyroid nodules are benign. Thyroid cancer is rare, accounting for only 1% of malignancies in the United States.

IMAGING RATIONALE
CT can detect thyroid nodules, but cannot characterize them. Ultrasound is the first line of imaging study for evaluation of a thyroid mass because

- It can determine if a palpable neck mass is in fact arising from the thyroid. Nonthyroidal neck masses include enlarged lymph nodes, aneurysms, and tumors arising from parathyroid, salivary glands, or muscle.
- The sonographic characteristics of a thyroid mass may provide an indication whether it is benign or malignant (for instance purely cystic lesions are always benign). However, pathognomonic signs of malignancy on sonography are unusual.
- Indeterminate lesions that are low suspicion for malignancy can be followed up with ultrasound to look for interval change. Those that are more suspicious can be biopsied with fine needle aspiration under sonographic guidance.

Tc99 isotope scan will distinguish "hot" (functioning) from "cold" (nonfunctioning) nodules. A hot nodule is more likely to be benign than a cold one, but 95% of thyroid nodules are cold. The Tc99 isotope scan is therefore of little value in distinguishing a benign from malignant thyroid nodule. Tc99 scan should be performed if thyroid function tests are abnormal as it is useful for diagnosing Graves' disease. Tc99 scan is also insensitive for detection of nodules 1 cm and smaller.

TEST OF CHOICE
Ultrasound, followed by ultrasound guided biopsy if needed.

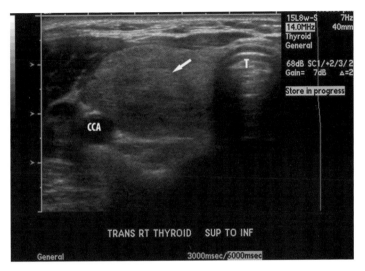

Figure 3-11   Axial ultrasound image of the neck shows right thyroid nodule (arrow). Trachea is marked with T and right carotid artery with CCA. CCA, common *carotid artery.*

BIBLIOGRAPHY

Feld S, Garcia M. AACE/AME Guidelines: American Association of Clinical Endocrinologists and Associazione Medici Endocrinologi Medical Guidelines for Clinical Practice for the Diagnosis and Management of Thyroid Nodules. American Association of Clinical Endocrinologists. 2006. Available at http://www.aace.com/pub/pdf/guidelines/thyroid_nodules.pdf.

Frates MC, Benson CB, Charboneau JW, et al. Management of thyroid nodules detected at US: Society of Radiologists in ultrasound consensus conference statement. *Radiology.* 2005;237:794-799.

4

DISEASES OF THE CHEST AND BREAST

Aamer R. Chughtai and
Wittaya Padungchaichote

4-1. Postoperative Shortness of Breath

CASE HISTORY
A 65-year-old female with acute onset of pleuritic chest pain and shortness of breath who had a recent hip replacement surgery.

BACKGROUND
Acute pulmonary embolism is associated with high morbidity and mortality, particularly in patients with risk factors such as recent surgery to pelvis or hip/knee replacement, long travel, **oral contraceptive pill** (OCP), pregnancy, hypercoagulable states, and a previous history of pulmonary embolism and deep vein thrombosis. The usual clinical presentation is with sudden onset of chest pain, shortness of breath and nonproductive cough. Hemoptysis may be present in some cases. While these symptoms are non-specific and may be absent in many patients, the diagnosis has to be made rapidly to prevent pulmonary infarction and even death.

TEST RATIONALE
In a patient with nonspecific symptoms of chest pain and dyspnea, a chest radiograph is obtained in the first instance to rule out pneumothorax, lobar pneumonia, or a pleural effusion that may explain the presenting symptoms. In other cases, however, pulmonary embolism remains the primary consideration. Until recently, nuclear medicine ventilation/perfusion (V/Q) scan was the mainstay for evaluation of pulmonary embolism, with invasive catheter pulmonary angiography as the gold standard or reference test. However, the presence of pulmonary disease and other comorbidities limit the diagnostic value of V/Q scanning. Over the past decade, contrast-enhanced computed tomography (CT) pulmonary angiography has emerged as the single most important imaging modality for the diagnosis of acute pulmonary embolism (see Figs. 4-1A, 4-1B, and 4-1C). It is readily available and the images are ready for review in a matter of minutes. The sensitivity and specificity of CT pulmonary angiography are 90%–100% and 89%–94% respectively, with a high negative predictive value of 98%–99%. It is now considered the new standard of care for the diagnosis of acute pulmonary embolism.

TEST OF CHOICE
CT pulmonary angiography.

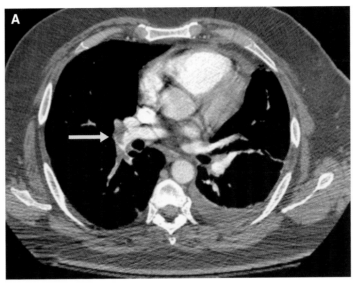

Figure 4-1 Contrast-enhanced CT pulmonary angiogram. Axial image (A) and coronal reconstruction (B) demonstrate an embolus in right lower lobe pulmonary artery (arrows). Delayed scan (C) through the thighs demonstrates a filling defect in right femoral vein consistent with deep vein thrombosis (arrow).
CT, computed tomography.

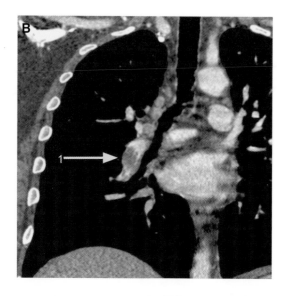

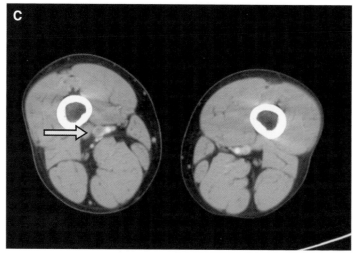

Figure 4-1 Continued.

BIBLIOGRAPHY
Baile EM, King GG, Muller NL, et al. Spiral computed tomography is comparable to angiography for the diagnosis of pulmonary embolism. *Am J Respir Crit Care Med.* 2000;161:1010-1015.
The PIOPED Investigators. Value of the ventilation/perfusion scan in acute pulmonary embolism. Results of the prospective investigation of pulmonary embolism diagnosis (PIOPED). *JAMA.* 1990;263:2753-2759.

4-2. Worsening Dyspnea with Joint Stiffness

CASE HISTORY
A 65-year-old female with worsening shortness of breath over last 1 year, history of pain and stiffness of joints of both hands.

BACKGROUND
Interstitial lung disease, such as idiopathic pulmonary fibrosis, can cause slowly progressing shortness of breath and fatigue. Idiopathic pulmonary fibrosis (IPF) should be suspected in patients with sarcoidosis, asbestosis, and many connective tissue disorders involving the lung, such as rheumatoid arthritis and scleroderma.

TEST RATIONALE
The interpretation of IPF on chest radiography can be very difficult; however, high-resolution CT accurately shows the true nature and extent of the interstitial process. Fortunately, the spectrum of CT features that suggest interstitial disease is small and includes interlobular septal thickening, honeycombing, nodules, traction bronchiectasis, and ground-glass opacification (see Figs. 4-2A and 4-2B). In IPF, which is the clinical diagnosis, the pattern seen on high-resolution CT is characteristic and is called usual interstitial pneumonitis. It includes architectural distortion, interlobular septal thickening, and honeycombing, particularly in peripheral lower lung distribution. These features are specific enough to obviate biopsy of the lung.

TEST OF CHOICE
High-resolution CT.

BIBLIOGRAPHY
Grenier P, Valeyre D, Cluzel P, Brauner MW, Lenoir S, Chastang C. Chronic diffuse interstitial lung disease: diagnostic value of chest radiography and high-resolution CT. *Radiology.* 1991;179(1):123-132.

Staples CA, Muller NL, Vedal S, Abboud R, Ostrow D, Miller RR. Usual interstitial pneumonia: correlation of CT with clinical, functional, and radiologic findings. *Radiology.* 1987;162(2):377-381.

Wells A. Clinical usefulness of high resolution computed tomography in cryptogenic fibrosing alveolitis. *Thorax.* 1998;53(12):1080-1087.

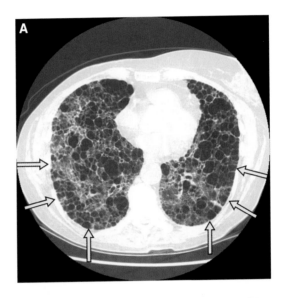

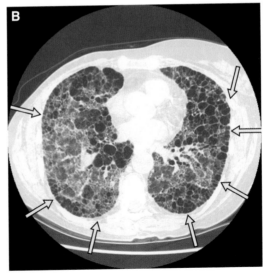

Figures 4-2 (A and B) Usual interstitial pneumonitis (UIP). High-resolution CT images through the mid and lower thorax demonstrate honeycomb cysts (arrows). Peripheral interlobular septal thickening and patchy ground-glass opacities are also present. CT, computed tomography.

4-3. Hypertension and Chest Pain

CASE HISTORY
A 70-year-old male with known hypertension presents with sudden-onset of tearing chest pain radiating to the back.

BACKGROUND
Aortic dissection is two to five times more common in men than women. By far the most important risk factor for aortic dissection is hypertension. Other risk factors include pregnancy, bicuspid aortic valve, Marfan's syndrome, Ehlers–Danlos syndrome, and trauma. It is important to recognize the possibility of aortic dissection in any patient presenting with sudden-onset tearing chest pain and promptly obtain appropriate imaging for definitive diagnosis.

TEST RATIONALE
A chest radiograph is usually the first imaging performed in a patient presenting with chest pain. It may show indirect signs of aortic pathology, such as a widened mediastinum, irregular aortic contour, deviation of the trachea or a nasogastric tube in the esophagus, and displacement of intimal calcification. However, chest radiograph is nonspecific and does not confirm the diagnosis. Historically, invasive catheter aortography was the definitive diagnostic modality; however, computed tomographic angiography has now replaced it as the new standard of care in imaging of the aorta (see Figs. 4-3A–F). It is noninvasive with high accuracy (99%), sensitivity (100%), and specificity (100%) for the diagnosis of aortic dissection. Patients unable to receive intravenous iodinated contrast can be evaluated with magnetic resonance imaging (MRI) of the aorta, which is also an accurate and noninvasive technique for examining patients suspected of having aortic dissection.

TESTS OF CHOICE
CT angiography; magnetic resonance angiography.

BIBLIOGRAPHY
Hayter RG, Rhea JT, Small A, Tafazoli FS, Novelline RA. Suspected aortic dissection and other aortic disorders: multi-detector row CT in 373 cases in the emergency setting. *Radiology.* 2006;238(3):841-852.

Jagannath AS, Sos TA, Lockhart SH, Saddekni S, Sniderman KW. Aortic dissection: a statistical analysis of the usefulness of plain chest radiographic findings. *AJR Am J Roentgenol.* 1986;147(6):1123-1126.

Nienaber CA, Eagle KA. Aortic dissection: new frontiers in diagnosis and management: Part I: from etiology to diagnostic strategies. *Circulation.* 2003;108(5):628-635.

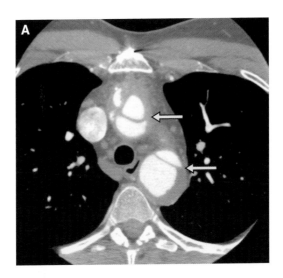

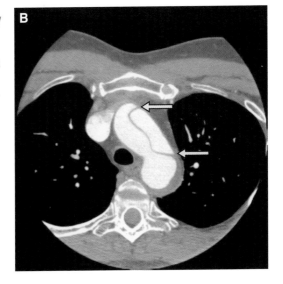

Figure 4-3 Selected axial (A and B) and coronal reformations (C and D) of contrast-enhanced CT angiography demonstrate a dissection flap in ascending and descending thoracic aorta (arrows), consistent with a type A aortic dissection. Gadolinium-enhanced axial SSFSE (E) and sagittal oblique cine balance gradient echo images (F) demonstrate a type B aortic dissection originating just distal to the left subclavian artery (arrows).
CT, computed tomography; SSFSE, single-shot fast spin-echo sequence

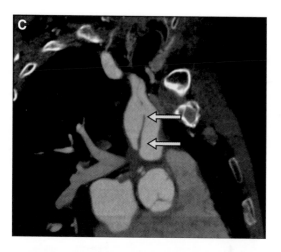

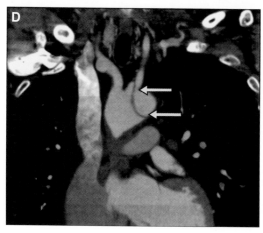

Figure 4-3 Continued.

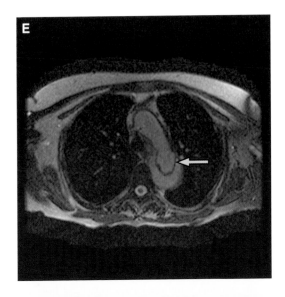

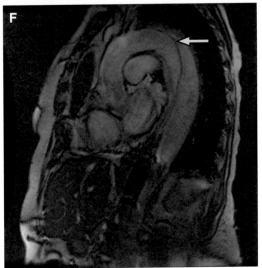

Figure 4-3 Continued.

4-4. Severe Central Chest Pain

CASE HISTORY

A 60-year-old male presents in the ER with sudden onset of central chest pain that has lasted for 3 minutes. The pain is relieved by rest. The patient has a history of 60 pack-year of smoking.

BACKGROUND

Chest pain is a common complaint with which more than 5 million people present to the ER every year. A significant number of these patients have acute coronary syndrome, which has to be diagnosed and managed emergently to reduce morbidity and mortality. The recognized risk factors of acute coronary syndrome include smoking, male gender, hypertension, diabetes mellitus, hyperlipidemia, and family history of coronary artery disease. The clinical signs and symptoms are nonspecific such as chest pain, nausea, shortness of breath, fatigue, and diaphoresis.

TEST RATIONALE

Many patients with chest pain may have noncardiac and/or nonemergent etiologies. A diagnostic test with a high negative predictive value for coronary artery disease that can also exclude other life-threatening causes of chest pain, such as pulmonary embolism and aortic dissection, could result in more efficient and cost-effective triage for patients presenting to the ER. There is now growing evidence that ECG-gated multislice coronary CT angiography may be that test (see Figs. 4-4A–D).

TEST OF CHOICE

Coronary CT angiography.

BIBLIOGRAPHY

Sato Y, Matsumoto N, Ichikawa M, et al. Efficacy of multislice computed tomography for the detection of acute coronary syndrome in the emergency department. *Circ J.* 2005;69(9):1047-1051.

White C, Read K, Kuo D. Assessment of chest pain in the emergency room: what is the role of multidetector CT? *Eur J Radiol.* 2006;57(3): 368-372.

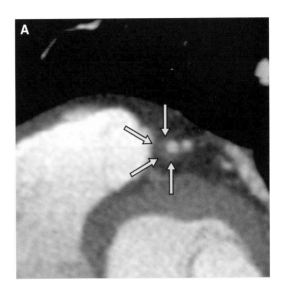

Figure 4-4 Coronary CT angiogram. Axial image (A) and multiplanar reformats (C and D) demonstrate a crescent of low attenuation material in the wall of left anterior descending coronary artery consistent with a noncalcified plaque (arrows). A multiplanar reformation (B) demonstrates a mixed calcified and noncalcified plaque in the left anterior descending coronary artery (arrows). CT, computed tomography.

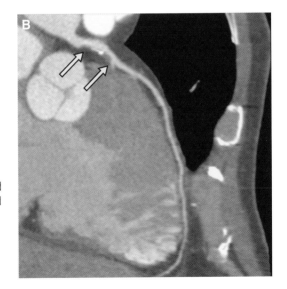

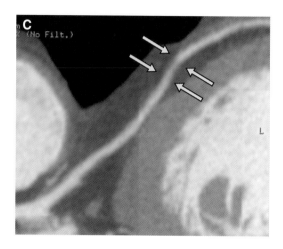

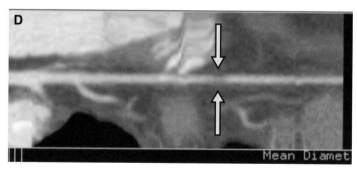

Figure 4-4   Continued.

4-5. Hemoptysis

CASE HISTORY
A 67-year-old male presents with weight loss and worsening cough over the past 4 months. He has now had three episodes of hemoptysis, and he is a heavy smoker.

BACKGROUND
Lung cancer remains the biggest killer among cancers with equal incidence in men and women, particularly in smokers. Other risk factors include asbestos, marijuana, radiation therapy to the lungs, and diseases causing scarring, such as tuberculosis. The symptoms can be nonspecific and include fatigue, shortness of breath, and weight loss. More specific symptoms include worsening long-term cough and hemoptysis. Lung cancer may begin as small nodules, and if detected early, they can be surgically resected. However, symptomatic patients may already have advanced disease that may not be curable.

TEST RATIONALE
In a smoker, symptoms such as weight loss and worsening cough, particularly with hemoptysis, should alert one to the possibility of lung cancer. Chest radiograph will show most of the larger masses (see Fig. 4-5A); however, smaller lesions (particularly central masses without obstructive signs) may go undetected. If such a lesion is suspected, CT of the chest will show the lesion and its extent (see Figs. 4-5B–D). However, use of CT screening for lung cancer is not recommended at present.

TEST OF CHOICE
Contrast-enhanced CT scan.

BIBLIOGRAPHY
Bach PB, Silvestri GA, Hanger M, Jett JR. Screening for lung cancer: ACCP evidence-based clinical practice guidelines (2nd edition). *Chest.* 2007;132(Suppl 3):69S-77S.

Thun MJ, Henley SJ, Burns DM, Jemal A, Shanks TG, Calle EE. Lung cancer death rates in lifelong nonsmokers. *J Natl Cancer Inst.* 2006;98(10):691-699.

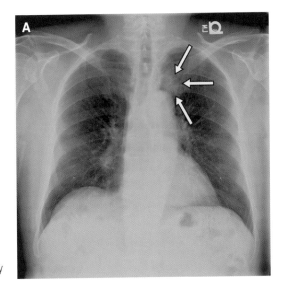

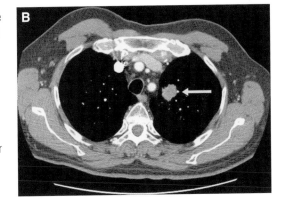

Figure 4-5   Frontal chest x-ray (A) demonstrates a nodular opacity in left upper lung medially (arrows). Selected-axial CT images through the upper chest on soft tissue (B) and lung windows (C) demonstrate a lobulated mass in left upper lobe consistent with a primary bronchogenic carcinoma (arrows). A right adrenal metastasis (arrow) is noted on the section through the upper abdomen (D). CT, computed tomography.

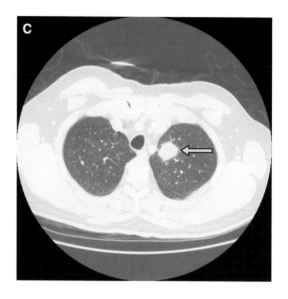

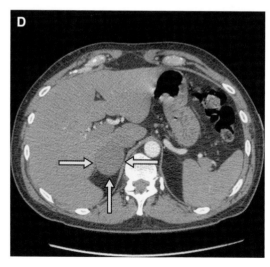

Figure 4-5 Continued.

4-6. Progressive Shortness of Breath

CASE HISTORY
A 75-year-old man presents with history of progressive shortness of breath, fatigue, and cough over the past year. He has been breeding birds since retirement.

BACKGROUND
Chronic hypersensitivity pneumonitis should be considered in patients who present with chronic or recurrent cough and shortness of breath or a history of recurrent episodes of acute respiratory symptoms without definite infectious triggers, particularly in a patient living in close proximity to birds. Other risk factors for chronic hypersensitivity pneumonitis include exposure to organic materials such as moldy hay, straw, and other organic dust, use of hot tub, presence of fungus in heating and cooling systems. To diagnose chronic hypersensitivity pneumonitis, a high index of suspicion and a comprehensive environmental history are essential.

TEST RATIONALE
Hypersensitivity pneumonitis is an immunologic response occurring in the lung to repeated exposures to inhaled organic material. It manifests as reticulonodular opacities on the chest radiograph, later progressing to lung fibrosis and honeycombing. Ground-glass opacification may be present in acute cases (see Figs. 4-6A–D). These findings are nonspecific for chronic hypersensitivity pneumonitis; however, high-resolution CT (HRCT) has been shown to distinguish chronic hypersensitivity pneumonitis from idiopathic pulmonary fibrosis in most, but not in all cases.

TEST OF CHOICE
High-resolution chest CT.

BIBLIOGRAPHY
Lynch DA, Newell JD, Logan PM, King TE Jr, Muller NL. Can CT distinguish hypersensitivity pneumonitis from idiopathic pulmonary fibrosis? *AJR Am J Roentgenol.* 1995;165(4):807-811.

Reynolds HY. Hypersensitivity pneumonitis. *Clin Chest Med.* 1982;3(3):503-519.

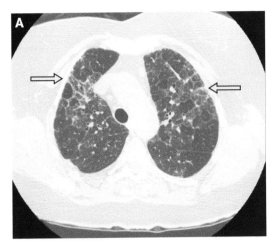

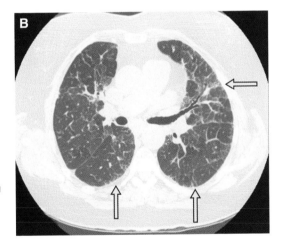

Figure 4-6 Chronic hypersensitivity pneumonitis. Selected high-resolution CT images through the upper and mid lungs (A, B, and C) demonstrate peripheral interlobular septal thickening, ground-glass opacities (arrows). A section through the lower lungs (D) demonstrates mosaic attenuation where the low attenuation areas represent lobules with air trapping.
CT, computed tomography.

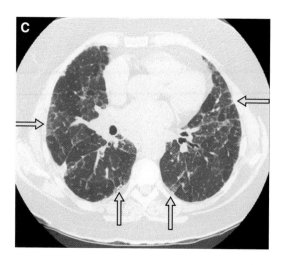

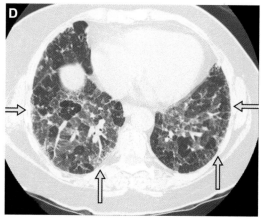

Figure 4-6 Continued.

4-7. Syncope, History of Malignancy

CASE HISTORY
A 45-year-old male with a 10-day history of significant shortness of breath, syncope, and fatigue. He has a history of resection of liposarcoma from left upper extremity 3 months ago.

BACKGROUND
Cardiac tumors can present with nonspecific symptoms such as progressive shortness of breath and fatigue. The majority of cardiac masses are metastases. Primary tumors of lung, breast, lymphomas, and melanomas are most likely to metastasize to the heart and pericardium. Primary cardiac tumors are mostly benign, such as myxomas and lipomas. The symptoms and signs of cardiac tumors depend on part of the heart affected. For example, a left atrial myxoma may cause obstruction to the flow of blood from the left atrium to the left ventricle. There may be enlargement of heart, murmurs, and arrythmias.

TEST RATIONALE
Clinically, the symptoms of cardiac and pericardial metastases are not characteristic and serious complications including stroke, myocardial infarction, and even sudden death from arrhythmia may be the first signs of tumor. When tumor involves the left ventricle, angina and dyspnea can be the presenting symptoms. Syncope can occur if the tumor involves the outflow tract. The diagnosis can be made initially with echocardiography; however, it is limited by several factors such as restricted field of view, body habitus, and blind spots. Cardiac CT and MRI are now more established techniques to diagnose, characterize, and examine the true extent of disease for treatment planning (see Figs. 4-7A–D).

TEST OF CHOICE
CT angiography and/or cardiac MRI.

BIBLIOGRAPHY
Butany J, Leong SW, Carmichael K, Komeda M. A 30-year analysis of cardiac neoplasms at autopsy. *Can J Cardiol.* 2005;21(8):675-680.

Fairman EB, Mauro VM, Cianciulli TF, et al. Liposarcoma causing left ventricular outflow tract obstruction and syncope: a case report and review of the literature. *Int J Cardiovasc Imaging.* 2005;21(5):513-518.

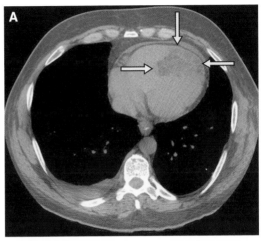

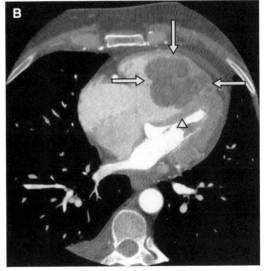

Figure 4-7 ECG-gated non–contrast-enhanced cardiac CT demonstrates a large lobulated low attenuation mass (of fat density) within the right ventricular cavity (A). ECG-gated axial contrast material enhanced cardiac CT (B) demonstrates deformity of the right ventricle walls and the interventricular septum (arrowhead). A coronal reconstruction (C) shows the mass occupying most of the right ventricle and breaching the right ventricular wall at the apex (arrowhead) and extends superiorly into the pulmonary outflow tract on a sagittal reconstruction (D). CT, computed tomography; ECG, electrocardiogram.

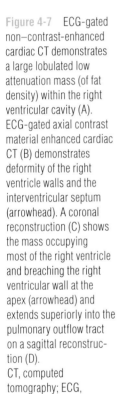

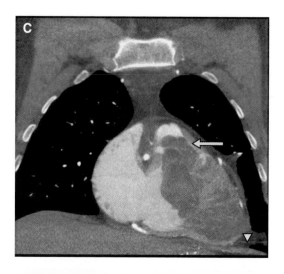

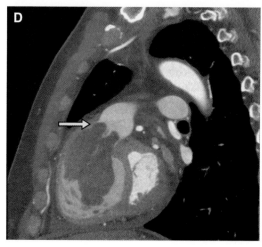

Figure 4-7 Continued.

4-8. Chest Trauma

CASE HISTORY
A 18-year-old male, brought to ER via survival flight with a history of motor vehicle accident (MVA).

BACKGROUND
MVAs are the leading cause of major chest trauma, particularly in young adults. The role of radiology in evaluation and management of chest trauma is complex and multifaceted. The symptoms depend on the type of chest trauma, for example, a hemodynamically unstable patient may have major vessel injury, such as aortic rupture. A tension pneumothorax or a large hemothorax/effusion may be present in patient with shortness of breath and decreasing oxygen saturation. The goal is to obtain all clinically important information rapidly and efficiently, which can be achieved with prompt imaging of the chest.

TEST RATIONALE
Chest trauma could either be penetrating, where chest wall integrity is breached, or be blunt, where the chest wall remains intact. The chest radiograph is one of the most important radiographic examinations as a rapid triage tool, however, CT is a more accurate and now rapidly available tool to characterize thoracic injuries, particularly of the thoracic aorta. Early diagnosis of thoracic aortic injury is important because prompt and definitive treatment can decrease mortality (see Figs. 4-8A and 4-8B). The reported negative predictive value of multidetector CT for diagnosis of aortic injuries has been 100% with a specificity of 96% when using direct signs of injury. Multidetector CT can now be performed within minutes of the patient's arrival in the ER, effectively eliminating other time consuming and more invasive diagnostic modalities.

TEST OF CHOICE
Contrast-enhanced CT scan with reformatted images of the spine and aorta.

BIBLIOGRAPHY
Scaglione M, Pinto A, Pinto F, Romano L, Ragozzino A, Grassi R. Role of contrast-enhanced helical CT in the evaluation of acute thoracic aortic injuries after blunt chest trauma. *Eur Radiol.* 2001;11(12):2444-2448.

Sinclair DS. Traumatic aortic injury: an imaging review. *Emerg Radiol.* 2002;9(1):13-20.

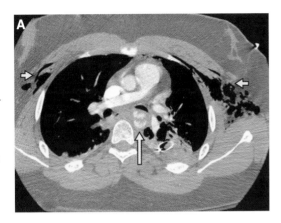

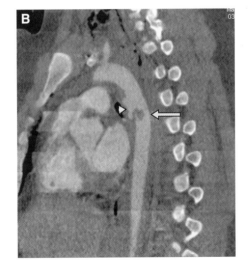

Figure 4-8 Axial contrast-enhanced CT image at the level of right pulmonary artery (A) demonstrates interruption in the continuity of the proximal descending thoracic aorta representing traumatic aortic rupture (long arrow). Subcutaneous emphysema is present in anterior and lateral chest wall (short arrows). A Sagittal reconstruction (B) demonstrates the traumatic dissection (long arrow) and a pseudoaneurysm in the proximal descending thoracic aorta (arrowhead). The aorta is relatively immobile just distal to the ligamentum arteriosum, making it susceptible to rupture at this point secondary to sudden deceleration during trauma. CT, computed tomography.

4-9. Shortness of Breath

CASE HISTORY
A 21-year-old man presents with sudden shortness of breath.

BACKGROUND
Spontaneous pneumothorax occurs in otherwise healthy young adults without any history of preexisting lung disease. The patient usually presents with sudden onset of chest pain. There may be prior history of similar episodes. On examination, the breath sounds may be absent on the side with suspected pneumothorax, there may be tracheal shift and hyperresonance on percussion. It is therefore easy to diagnose; however, in recurrent episodes, an attempt to look for potential cause can be useful to treat and prevent further recurrences.

TEST RATIONALE
Most pneumothoraces can be easily seen on a chest radiograph (see Fig. 4-9A). However, when searching for a cause of pneumothorax, such as apical blebs, CT of the chest has been shown to be very sensitive (see Figs. 4-9B and 4-9C). This information is very useful in treatment planning and preventing further recurrences.

TEST OF CHOICE.
Non–contrast-enhanced chest CT.

BIBLIOGRAPHY
Fiore D, Biondetti PR, Sartori F, Calabró F. The role of computed tomography in the evaluation of bullous lung disease. *J Comput Assist Tomogr.* 1982;6(1):105-108.

Warner BW, Bailey WW, Shipley RT. Value of computed tomography of the lung in the management of primary spontaneous pneumothorax. *Am J Surg.* 1991;162(1):39-42.

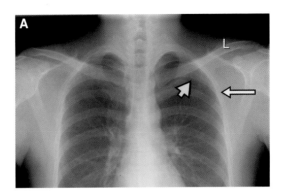

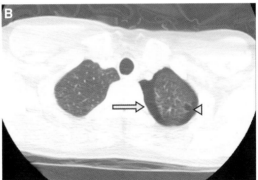

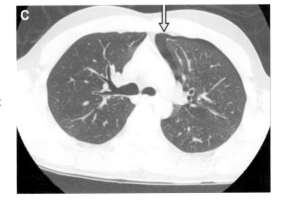

Figure 4-9
Spontaneous pneumothorax. Frontal chest radiograph (A) demonstrates a left pneumothorax (long arrow). A pleural edge is seen (short arrow). Axial chest CT images through upper and mid chest with lung windows (B and C) demonstrate a left apical pneumothorax (long arrows). In addition, there is a small bleb in left apex with interruption of its lateral wall (arrowhead), likely cause of the pneumothorax.
CT, computed tomography.

4-10. Fever and Chest Pain

CASE HISTORY
A 46-year-old female presents with right upper quadrant pain, high-grade fever, and chills.

BACKGROUND
Right upper quadrant pain with fever in a middle-aged female is usually an indicator of acute gall bladder pathology; however, right lower lobe pneumonia can present with similar symptoms. A chest radiograph here would be a quick and easy way to confirm the diagnosis.

TEST RATIONALE
The diagnosis of pneumonia can be made with clinical assessment and confirmed with radiological imaging. The initial investigation of choice in a patient suspected of lobar pneumonia would be a chest radiograph (see Figs. 4-10A and 4-10B). It is readily available and therefore commonly used because of its high cost–benefit ratio. The patient can then be followed up with chest radiographs after antibiotic therapy (see Fig. 4-10C). If the infection is persistent or when complications of pneumonia are suspected, CT of the chest can be used to evaluate the extent of infection and to detect predisposing factors.

TEST OF CHOICE
Chest radiograph; Contrast-enhanced chest CT.

BIBLIOGRAPHY
Van Mieghem IM, De Wever WF, Verschakelen JA. Lung infection in radiology: a summary of frequently depicted signs. *Jbr-Btr.* 2005;88(2):66-71.
Vilar J, Domingo ML, Soto C, Cogollos J. Radiology of bacterial pneumonia. *Eur J Radiol.* 2004;51(2):102-113.

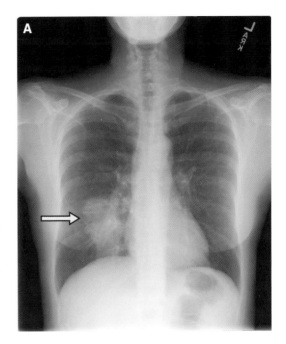

Figure 4-10   Frontal (A) and lateral (B) chest radiographs demonstrate a large opacity in the middle lobe (arrows) in keeping with pneumonia. Follow-up chest radiograph (C) after 6 weeks shows complete resolution of pneumonia.

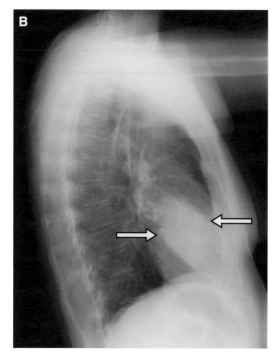

Figure 4-10 Continued.

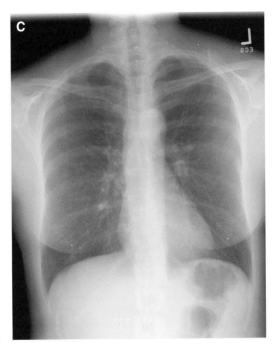

Figure 4-10 Continued.

4-11. Dysphagia

CASE HISTORY

A 61-year-old female presented approximately 1 year ago with symptoms of musculoskeletal type chest pain and weakness. She now complains of intermittent sensations of neck fullness, swelling, and dysphagia. She underwent a CT chest demonstrating an anterior mediastinal mass. This was resected and shown to be a thymoma on pathology.

BACKGROUND

Thymomas are relatively less common than other tumors arising in the anterior mediastinum, namely, malignant lymphoma, mature teratoma, and thyroid masses. Other thymic tumors that can be considered in the differential include thymic carcinoma and thymic endocrine tumors.

Clinical differentiation of these tumors is important as the treatment and management is different for each. Thymomas can present with nonspecific clinical symptoms of dyspnea and chest fullness; however, one-third of patients can develop myasthenia gravis with more specific symptoms such as blurred vision, weakness, and dysphagia. Surgical resection is the preferred choice for thymoma, whereas in lymphomas or other nonthymic tumors, a biopsy may be appropriate for tissue diagnosis.

TEST RATIONALE

CT and MRI are the preferred methods to image the thymus and to differentiate it from other anterior mediastinal masses (see Fig. 4-11). CT can demonstrate the extent of tumor, nodal involvement, and metastases. CT has been shown to be equal or superior to MRI in the diagnosis of the majority of anterior mediastinal masses.

TEST OF CHOICE

Contrast-enhanced CT of the chest.

BIBLIOGRAPHY

Drachman DB. Myasthenia gravis. N Engl J Med. 1994;330(25):1797-1810.

Srirajaskanthan R, Toubanakis C, Dusmet M, Caplin ME. A review of thymic tumours. Lung Cancer. 2008;60(1):4-13.

Tomiyama N, Honda O, Tsubamoto M, et al. Anterior mediastinal tumors: diagnostic accuracy of CT and MRI. Eur J Radiol. 2009 Feb;69(2): 280-288.

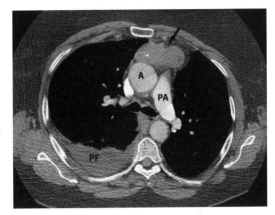

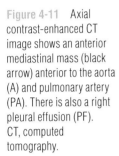

Figure 4-11 Axial contrast-enhanced CT image shows an anterior mediastinal mass (black arrow) anterior to the aorta (A) and pulmonary artery (PA). There is also a right pleural effusion (PF). CT, computed tomography.

4-12. Painful Breast Mass

CASE HISTORY
A 26-year-old lactating woman presented with a painful palpable mass in the left breast.

BACKGROUND
Lactational breast infection is a common condition for 9% of puerperal women. The patient usually has painful red swollen breast associated with fever. The local signs of infection vary greatly with the stage of infection and range from mild cellulitis to an abscess. In early cases (mastitis) surgery is meddlesome and unnecessarily destructive. Whereas, continued antibiotic therapy in the presence of an abscess may lead to unnecessary tissue destruction by the disease process.

Other conditions presenting with a palpable tender mass include fibrocystic changes, galactocele, fat necrosis, plasma cell mastitis (duct ectasia), and superficial thrombophlebitis (Mondor's disease). Inflammatory breast cancer can cause swelling and redness of the breast but is rarely painful and is uncommon in young patients.

TEST RATIONALE
Ultrasound is the imaging modality of choice in evaluating breast abnormalities for young women (under 30), lactating women, and pregnant women (see Fig. 4-12A). Ultrasound is also used in the guidance of interventional procedures such as aspiration, abscess drainage, biopsy, and wire localization.

Mammography is less effective in younger women because of the greater dense breast tissue that lowers the sensitivity of the mammogram. However, if ultrasound identifies a suspicious abnormality, mammography should be performed to identify possible multifocal lesions or an intraductal component of an invasive tumor (see Fig. 4-12B).

TEST OF CHOICE
Ultrasound with/without mammograms.

BIBLIOGRAPHY
Bassett LW. Imaging of breast masses. *Radiol Clin North Am.* 2000;38(4):669-691.
Mendelson EB. Problem-solving ultrasound. *Radiol Clin North Am.* 2004;42(5):909-918.

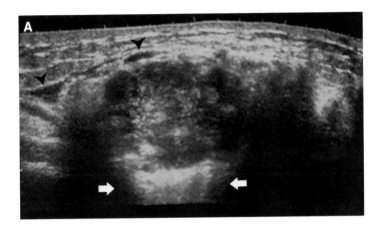

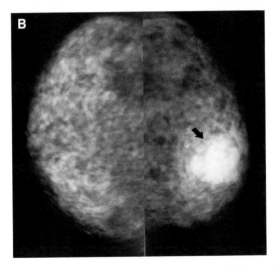

Figure 4-12   Abscess in a 26-year-old woman with a palpable painful mass in the left breast. (A) Panoramic US image of the left breast (7 o'clock position) shows a partially circumscribed, lobulated, inhomogeneous hypoechoic mass with posterior enhancement (white arrows). There is edema of premammary fat (black arrowheads). (B) Bilateral CC mammograms show a partially circumscribed, partially obscured (arrow), lobulated mass in the inner quadrant of the left breast.
CC, craniocaudal; US, ultrasound.

4-13. Painless Breast Mass

CASE HISTORY
A 55-year-old woman presents with a palpable painless mass in the left breast.

BACKGROUND
Breast cancer is the second most common cancer and the second leading cause of cancer deaths for American women. Although at least 75% of palpable breast mass are benign, breast cancer must be included in the differential diagnosis of any breast mass. Risk factors of breast cancer include age, age at menarche, age at first live birth, history of previous breast cancer, ovarian cancer, endometrial cancer, history of first-degree relative with breast cancer, race (white women have greater risk than black women), and obesity.

TEST RATIONALE
Diagnostic mammography is indicated in patients age 30 or older when there are clinical findings, such as a palpable mass, localized pain or nipple discharge. An abnormal screening mammogram also requires additional work-up. Management of the patient may change depending on the mammogram. The benefits of mammography include demonstrating that the palpable abnormality is benign and avoidance of further intervention (calcified involuting fibroadenoma, lipoma, oil cyst, galactocele, or hamartoma); reinforcing the impression that the palpable abnormality is likely malignant and supporting earlier intervention; ability to search the remainder of the ipsilateral breast and contralateral breast for clinically occult cancer and assess the extent of a malignancy and multifocality when cancer is diagnosed (see Fig. 4-13A).

Breast ultrasound remains the most cost effective, accurate, and useful of the adjunctive breast imaging tools and is available in virtually every practice. It is clearly the instrument of choice for image-guided breast biopsies and preoperative needle localizations and has revolutionized diagnostic breast evaluation by providing rapid, inexpensive, and accurate guidance for breast intervention (see Fig. 4-13B).

A negative mammogram and/or ultrasound should not defer the biopsy of a clinically suspicious finding.

TEST OF CHOICE
Diagnostic mammography with/without breast ultrasound.

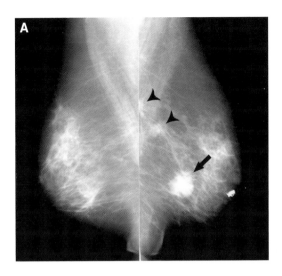

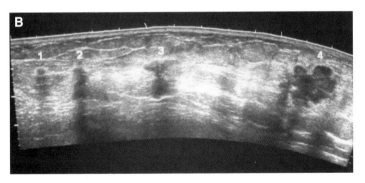

Figure 4-13 Multicentric breast cancers in a 55-year-old woman with a palpable mass in the left breast. (A) Bilateral MLO mammograms show a dominant spiculated mass (arrow; at palpable site) in left lower quadrant and two smaller spiculated masses (arrowheads, nonpalpable) in left upper quadrant. (B) Panoramic US image of the left breast scanned from LUOQ through LLIQ shows four irregular solid masses. The biggest mass (4) is palpable. The mass (1) is not included in the left MLO mammogram. LLIQ, left lower inner quadrant; LUOQ, left lower outer quadrant; MLO, mediolateral oblique; US, ultrasound.

BIBLIOGRAPHY

Kopans DB. Evaluating women with lumps, thickening, discharge, or pain: imaging women with signs or symptoms that might indicate breast cancer. In: Kopans DB, ed. *Breast imaging.* 3rd ed. Philadelphia: Lippincott Williams & Wilkins; 2006:733-751.

Yang W, Dempsey PJ. Diagnostic breast ultrasound: current status and future directions. *Radiol Clin North Am.* 2007;45(5):845-861.

5

DISEASES OF THE GASTROINTESTINAL TRACT

Julia R. Fielding and Wui K. Chong

5-1. Crohn Disease

CASE HISTORY
A 25-year-old male presents with recurrent bouts of right lower quadrant pain and diarrhea.

BACKGROUND
Crohn disease is an autoimmune process that involves the bowel and other organs. Symptoms include the classic abdominal pain, episodic diarrhea, perianal pain due to fistula and occasionally fever. In most cases, the disease presents before the age of 30. Diagnosis is made using colonoscopy with biopsy of involved segments of the large and small bowel. The terminal ileum is the most common site of disease; however, any portion of the gastrointestinal tract may be involved. Once a patient has been diagnosed, recurrent bouts of disease with complications including fistulae and abscess are common.

TEST RATIONALE
The initial presentation of Crohn disease is similar to appendicitis and infectious colitis and ileitis. Computed tomography (CT) scan is performed to identify circumferential bowel wall thickening, skip areas, tethering of bowel loops, and presence of abscess, which are nearly diagnostic of the disease (see Figs. 5-1A and 5-1B). The identification of abscess is particularly important as it may require percutaneous drainage. Long-term follow-up of small-bowel disease is usually performed using a fluoroscopic small bowel follow-through to identify areas of stricture and obstruction. Clinical suspicion of abscess may require repeat CT scan. In the future, magnetic resonance imaging (MRI) may be employed to diminish the cumulative effects of radiation.

TEST OF CHOICE
CT scan.

BIBLIOGRAPHY
Goldberg HI, Gore RM, Margulis AR, Moss AA, Baker EL. Computed tomography in the evaluation of Crohn disease. *AJR Am J Roentgenol.* 1983 Feb;140(2):277-282.

Jaffe TA, Gaca AM, Delaney S, et al. Radiation doses from small-bowel follow-through and abdominopelvic MDCT in Crohn's disease. *AJR Am J Roentgenol.* 2007 Nov;189(5):1015-1022.

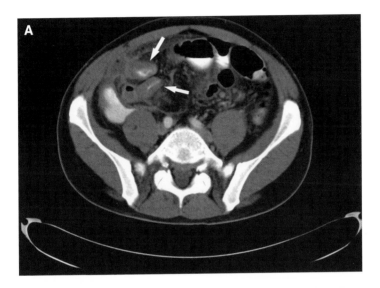

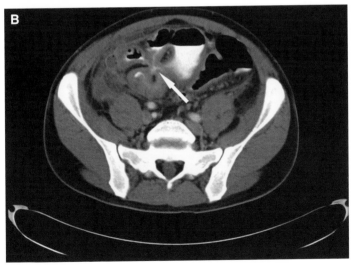

Figure 5-1 (A) Axial CT scan of the pelvis show two thick-walled loops of bowel in the right lower quadrant (arrows). (B) Scan inferior that in (A) shows an enteroenteric fistulae (arrows), a common complication.
CT, computed tomography.

5-2. Dropping Hematocrit

CASE HISTORY
A 61-year-old male becomes diaphoretic and tachycardic 2 hours following angiogram.

BACKGROUND
Many patients presenting with ischemic cardiac symptomatology will undergo catheterization as part of diagnosis and treatment. In most cases, a catheter is introduced via the groin into the iliac artery and extended cephalad to the coronary sinus. Contrast material is injected to identify stenoses of the coronary arteries that might be the cause of angina or infarction. In some cases, treatment using coronary artery stents is performed at the time of the procedure. Many of these patients receive blood thinning drugs, such as heparin, before and during the procedure to avoid clot formation. This increases the risk of a postprocedure hemorrhage, which occurs in approximately 2% of cases.

TEST RATIONALE
A patient with an active hemorrhage must be assessed immediately. The fastest and the most accurate test is a non–contrast-enhanced CT scan (see Figs. 5-2A and 5-2B). Most postcatheterization hemorrhages occur along the course of the catheter and extend into the retroperitoneum and involve the psoas muscle. High density within the hematoma usually indicates active bleeding and may require urgent embolization or repair of the torn vessel.

TEST OF CHOICE
Non–contrast-enhanced CT scan.

BIBLIOGRAPHY
Ellis SG, Bhatt D, Kapadia S, Lee D, Yen M, Whitlow PL. Correlates and outcomes of retroperitoneal hemorrhage complicating percutaneous coronary intervention. *Catheter Cardiovasc Interv.* 2006 Apr;67(4): 541-545.

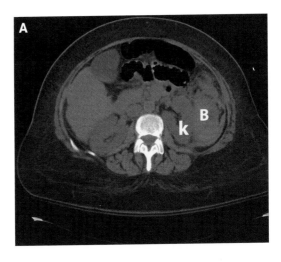

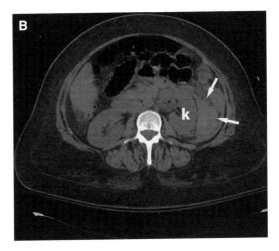

Figure 5-2 (A and B)
Axial images of the
midabdomen show the
left kidney (k), an adjacent
bowel loop (b) and an
ovoid bright hematoma
(arrows).

5-3. Palpable Abdominal Mass

CASE HISTORY
A 54-year-old obese female patient reports recent development of a painless mass near the umbilicus.

BACKGROUND
The abdominal organs are contained by a combination of the peritoneum, muscles, and fibrous condensations. Obese patients and those with a previous open abdominal surgery, particularly in the midline, often have a lax abdominal wall. Increasing obesity, chronic obstructive pulmonary disease, and lifting of heavy objects all contribute to the force placed on the abdominal wall. In some cases there is a tear or diastasis of the muscles, fibrous tissue, and peritoneum, and an abdominal wall hernia results. Hernias may contain fat or bowel. Common sites of hernias include the midline with separation of the linea alba, the inguinal canal, and the umbilicus. In many cases they are palpable but otherwise asymptomatic; however, hernias are usually repaired to avoid development of bowel or omental entrapment and strangulation.

TEST RATIONALE
In both the symptomatic and asymptomatic patient a non–contrast-enhanced CT scan is usually the first test performed. Although no intravenous contrast is necessary, oral contrast is essential to identify small and large bowel loops (see Figs. 5-3A and 5-3B). Once a hernia is diagnosed, findings must be reported for surgical planning. Specifically, the location of the hernia, the contents of the hernia, such as bowel, omentum, or abdominal organs, and the presence of adjacent vital organs are important facts in planning the optimal repair. In postoperative patients, fluid is often seen surrounding the mesh repair. Rim enhancement or gas bubbles indicate infection.

TEST OF CHOICE
Non–contrast-enhanced CT scan.

BIBLIOGRAPHY
Lin BH, Vargish T, Dachman AH. CT findings after laparoscopic repair of ventral hernia. *AJR Am J Roentgenol.* 1999 Feb;172(2):389-392.

MacKersie AB, Lane MJ, Gerhardt RT, et al. Nontraumatic acute abdominal pain: unenhanced helical CT compared with three-view acute abdominal series. *Radiology.* 2005 Oct(1);237:114-122.

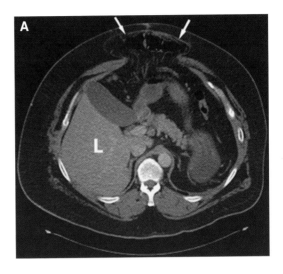

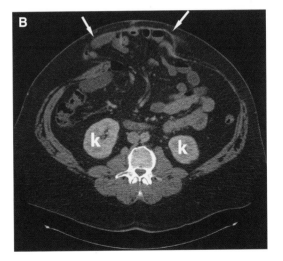

Figure 5-3 (A and B)
Axial images with the liver demarcated by L and kidneys with K. Arrows delineate the protruding peritoneum which contains a small bowel loop.

5-4. Dysphagia

CASE HISTORY
A 75-year-old female complains of difficulty swallowing solid food.

BACKGROUND
Dysphagia, difficulty swallowing, and odynophagia, painful swallowing are common problems, particularly in the elderly. Following a physical examination to exclude obvious problems, such as a visible oral or hypopharyngeal mass, most patients require evaluation of the esophagus. In some cases, especially those where biopsy is likely, this is performed with upper endoscopy. In others, indirect visualization is performed using a barium swallow. Because pain can be referred to locations beyond that of the disease, the entire esophagus must be imaged. The differential diagnosis includes stricture usually due to acid reflux, hernias, abnormal peristalsis, and neoplasms. Barium swallow is also extremely sensitive in detection of esophageal perforation into the chest.

TEST RATIONALE
The barium swallow is an inexpensive test that allows visualization of the entire esophagus in multiple planes. Images of the cervical esophagus may show hypertrophy of the cricopharyngeus, a posterior Zencker's diverticulum, or aspiration. Most strictures and tumors occur in the lower third of esophagus. In the case of impacted food, the barium swallow can detect perforation of the esophagus into the chest (see Fig. 5-4).

TEST OF CHOICE
Barium swallow.

BIBLIOGRAPHY
Prabhakar A, Levine MS, Rubesin S, L et al. Relationship between diffuse esophageal spasm and lower esophageal sphincter dysfunction on barium studies and manometry in 14 patients. *AJR Am J Roentgenol.* 2004 Aug;(2);183:409-413.

Swanson JO, Levine MS, Redfern RO, et al. Usefulness of high-density barium for detection of leaks after esophagogastrectomy, total gastrectomy, and total laryngectomy. *AJR Am J Roentgenol.* 2003 Aug;181 (2):415-420.

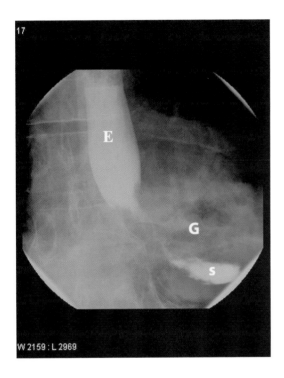

Figure 5-4 Normal appearing esophagus (E) empties into a small stomach (S). Irregular gas marks the site of a perforation (G).

5-5. Diverticulitis

CASE HISTORY
A 70-year-old female presents with left lower quadrant pain, fever, and diarrhea.

BACKGROUND
Left lower quadrant pain has a wide differential; however, in an elderly patient, diverticulitis should be considered as a likely source. Diverticula, small outpouchings of the colon, develop with age and are located primarily within the left and sigmoid portions of the colon. In most cases they are of no clinical significance. Occasionally, bowel contents become trapped inside a diverticulum with resulting inflammation of the wall and microperforation. Complications include ischemia, abscess, and pneumoperitoneum. Uncomplicated cases usually respond to antibiotics. Abscesses require drainage. Repeat episodes of diverticulitis are usually treated with sigmoid resection.

TEST RATIONALE
Contrast-enhanced CT scan shows the site of bowel abnormality and the presence of free air and fluid collections (see Fig. 5-5A). Classic findings include long-segment circumferential wall thickening of the colon with associated vascular engorgement and inflammation of the adjacent fat. Free air usually indicates a large perforation and may require urgent surgery. Other colonic pathologies that may mimic diverticulitis include colitis and perforated colon cancer. Colitis usually involves a long segment of the colon with massive wall thickening (see Fig. 5-5B). Colon cancer is most often short-segment disease with an associated mass and adjacent enlarged lymph nodes.

TEST OF CHOICE
Contrast-enhanced CT.

BIBLIOGRAPHY
Goh V, Halligan S, Taylor SA, Burling D, et al.. Differentiation between diverticulitis and colorectal cancer: quantitative CT perfusion measurements versus morphologic criteria—initial experience. *Radiology.* 2007 Feb;242(2):456-462.

Horton KM, Abrams RA, Fishman EK. Spiral CT of colon cancer: imaging features and role in management. *Radiographics.* 2000 March–April;20 (2):419-430.

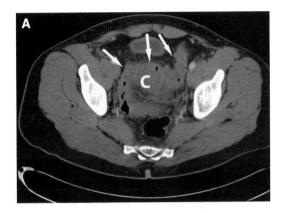

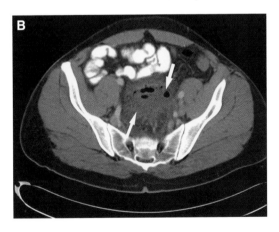

Figure 5-5 Axial image (A) shows dots of free air and fluid just superior to the colon indicative of abscess. Image (B) shows the thick-walled colon delineated by arrows.

5-6. Appendicitis

CASE HISTORY
A 25-year-old female presents with right lower quadrant pain, fever, and obstipation.

BACKGROUND
In the young male, the symptoms described earlier are nearly diagnostic of acute appendicitis. A surgeon will often take the patient to the operating room based on the history and physical examination alone. In the female patient, gynecologic pathology mimics that of acute appendicitis therefore imaging is often required. When the pelvic examination suggests the ovary as the source of pain, a transvaginal ultrasound (US) is indicated. If this test is negative, a contrast-enhanced CT scan is usually required before the patient goes to surgery. Regarding pediatric patients, US should be used as an abnormal appendix can be identified in the majority of cases.

TEST RATIONALE
Contrast-enhanced CT scan has exquisite depiction of the bowel. The appendix can be located in virtually all patients approximately 10 mm below the ileocecal valve, although it may extend superior, medial, or posterior to the cecum. A thick-walled tubular structure arising from the cecum and separate from the terminal ileum is diagnostic of appendicitis (see Figs. 5-6A and 5-6B). Free fluid is common. Free air indicates perforation and an adjacent contained fluid collection is an abscess.

TEST OF CHOICE
Contrast-enhanced CT scan.

BIBLIOGRAPHY
Jacobs JE, Birnbaum BA, Macari M, et al. Acute appendicitis: comparison of helical CT diagnosis focused technique with oral contrast material versus nonfocused technique with oral and intravenous contrast material. *Radiology.* 2001 Sep;220(3):683-690.
Paulson EK, Kalady MF, Pappas TN. Clinical practice. Suspected appendicitis. *N Engl J Med.* 2003 Jan;16;348(3):236-242.

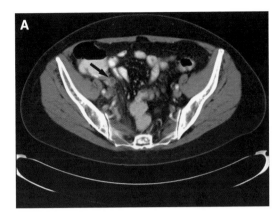

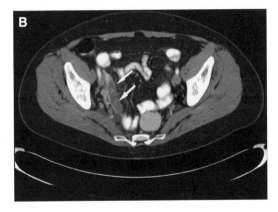

Figure 5-6   Axial image (A) shows a thick walled tubular and dilated appendix (white arrow). Image (B) shows the origin of the appendix adjacent to the cecum (black arrow).

5-7. Postoperative Fever

CASE HISTORY
A 45-year-old female presents with fever following sigmoid colon resection.

BACKGROUND
Many postoperative patients develop a fever within the first 48 hours following surgery. This is a common reaction and often resolves with improved lung aeration and mobility. When fever persists, the differential diagnosis includes the following: pneumonia, urinary tract infection from indwelling catheter, wound infection, drug reaction, and abscess. Abscess formation following pancreatic and bowel surgery may form within the first postoperative week.

TEST RATIONALE
Virtually all abscesses occur at or near the surgical site. Following abdominal surgery, pneumonia can often be excluded based on a chest radiograph. On contrast-enhanced CT scan, an abscess appears as a round or ovoid fluid collection, often with an enhancing rim. The presence of gas bubbles is less common but diagnostic (see Figs. 5-7A and 5-7B). The differential diagnosis includes hematoma and, depending on the surgical site, biloma or urinoma. CT and US can be used as guidance tools for percutaneous drainage.

TEST OF CHOICE
Contrast-enhanced CT of the abdomen and pelvis.

BIBLIOGRAPHY
Behrman SW, Zarzaur BL. Intra-abdominal sepsis following pancreatic resection: incidence, risk factors, diagnosis, microbiology, management, and outcome. *Am Surg.* 2008 Jul;74(7):572-578; Discussion 578-579.

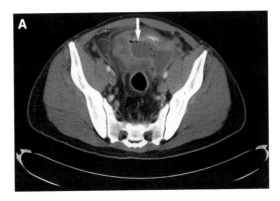

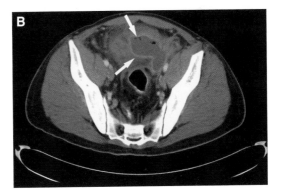

Figure 5-7 Arrows in figures (A) and (B) show the enhancing rim of a fluid collection that is outside of the bowel and contains dots of gas.

5-8. Small-Bowel Obstruction

CASE HISTORY
A 75-year-old male with a history of multiple abdominal surgeries presents with vomiting, abdominal distension and obstipation.

BACKGROUND
The most common causes for bowel obstruction include adhesions from previous surgery, incarcerated hernia, and metastases. The large bowel is rarely affected in adults likely because of its relatively short length and numerous fascial attachments to adjacent organs and the retroperitoneum. The small bowel is very long and mobile. Loops can extend to the peritoneum, the site of most adhesions, without difficulty. Adhesions may also occur near a surgical scar and in association with inflammatory bowel disease or radiation therapy. In a patient with a known cancer, metastases are a common cause of obstruction. An incarcerated hernia can be diagnosed on physical examination.

TEST RATIONALE
While CT scan has superseded the abdominal plain film for the diagnosis of the majority of serious abdominal diseases in the case of suspected small-bowel obstruction it should be performed as the initial test. Dilated loops of bowel with an abrupt transition point and minimal colonic gas are diagnostic of bowel obstruction (see Figs. 5-8A and 5-8B). Free air indicates a perforation and when associated with sepsis, may require immediate surgery. In addition, the uncommon large bowel obstruction can be identified. Once a small-bowel obstruction is identified on plain film, contrast-enhanced CT scan is performed to locate the site of obstruction and any associated soft tissue mass. In this case, oral contrast agents are not administered because the patient will be unable to tolerate additional fluid.

TEST OF CHOICE
Plain radiograph followed by contrast-enhanced CT of the abdomen and pelvis.

BIBLIOGRAPHY
Maglinte DD, Balthazar EJ, Kelvin FM, et al. The role of radiology in diagnosis of small-bowel obstruction. *AJR Am J Roentgenol.* 1997 May;168(5):1171-1180.

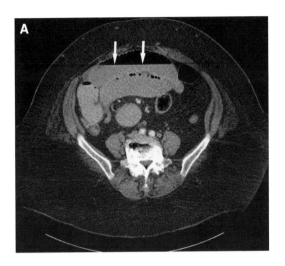

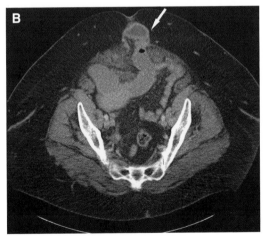

Figure 5-8 In axial image (A) Dilated small bowel loop contains dilute oral-contrast agent forming an air fluid level (arrows). (B) Shows the source of the small-bowel obstruction, a midline hernia containing a loop of small bowel (arrow). Note that small bowel loop within the left pelvis is not dilated and distal to the obstruction.

Paulson EK, Kalady MF, Pappas TN. Clinical practice. Suspected appendicitis. *N Engl J Med*. 2003 Jan;15;348(3):236-242.

Thompson WM, Kilani RK, Smith BB, et al. Accuracy of abdominal radiography in acute small-bowel obstruction: does reviewer experience matter? *AJR Am J Roentgenol*. 2007 Mar;188(3):W233-W238.

5-9. Solitary Liver Lesion

CASE HISTORY
A 49-year-old female with a history of breast cancer undergoes US for epigastric pain. No source for pain is identified; however, a single solid liver lesion is seen.

BACKGROUND
As more and more people undergo imaging, the aforementioned scenario has become common. The goal is to avoid further testing when possible while identifying those lesions that are suspicious for malignancy. In those patients with no known primary tumor, a cystic or solid liver lesion is rarely, if ever, malignant. If the lesion has no suspicious features on the US examination, a reasonable approach is no additional testing. If the patient has an unusual or complicated medical history, a repeat US can be performed in 6 months time to assure stability. In the case of a patient with known cancer, all liver lesions require additional imaging or biopsy to exclude metastases. Up to 60% of such lesions will be malignant neoplasms.

TEST RATIONALE
Contrast-enhanced CT, contrast-enhanced MRI, and positron emission tomography (PET) scans are sensitive and specific tests for the identification of liver metastases. Metastases are supplied by the hepatic arteries. The majority of lesions are solid masses with poorly defined borders that enhance brightly on arterial phase images (see Figs. 5-9A and 5-9B). Adenocarcinoma often has a lobulated contour. PET scans are very sensitive for the presence of malignancy because increased tracer uptake implies increased glucose consumption by the growing tumor. MRI rivals the sensitivity and specificity of PET and provides anatomic information for treatment. It is particularly useful in cases where there is baseline liver disease, such as cirrhosis. CT scan is less sensitive but more widely available. In the future, evaluation of most liver masses suspicious for malignant neoplasm will likely be performed using a combination of PET and CT or MRI.

TEST OF CHOICE
Dependent on patient history and availability of technology; in this case, MRI was performed.

BIBLIOGRAPHY
Bipat S, van Leeuwen MS, Comans EF, et al. Colorectal liver metastases: CT, MR imaging, and PET for diagnosis—met-analysis. *Radiology*. 2005 Oct;237(1):123-131. Epub 2005 Aug 11.

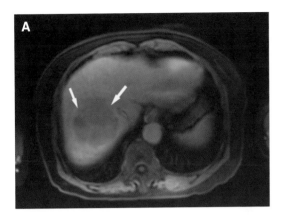

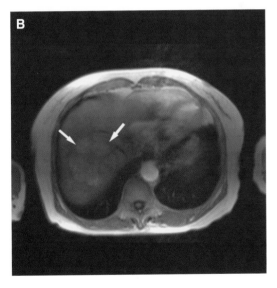

Figure 5-9 Two images from an MR series show a round lesion within the right lobe of the liver (arrows). Note the enhancing rim in image (A) and irregular enhancement of the mass in (B). MR, magnetic resonance.

Kamel IR, Choti MA, Horton KM, et al. Surgically staged focal liver lesions: accuracy and reproducibility of dual-phase helical CT for detection and characterization. *Radiology.* 2003 Jun;227(3):752-757.

5-10. Incomplete Colonoscopy

CASE HISTORY
A 60-year-old male with a history of colon cancer undergoes endoscopy. Because of the tortuosity of the colon, the ascending portion is not seen.

BACKGROUND
Virtual colonoscopy is a relatively new technology that uses non–contrast-enhanced CT scans to identify colonic polyps. At present, baseline colonoscopy is performed at age 50. In those patients with polyps, a repeat colonoscopy in 5 years is recommended. Some patients, especially the elderly have a long, looped colon that makes complete evaluation of the cecum and right colon impossible. In these patients, an additional test is required. This was usually a fluoroscopic barium enema. Virtual colonoscopy may soon replace this test.

TEST RATIONALE
Following a standard bowel cleansing protocol, the patient's colon is filled with CO_2. CT images are obtained in the supine and prone position. The examination for the patient is then complete. Software programs reconstruct the colon so that a virtual fly-through can be performed. Masses seen on the 3D reconstructions are correlated with axial images (see Figs. 5-10A and 5-10B). Pathology beyond the confines of the colon, such as enlarged lymph nodes and liver masses, can also be identified. In recent studies, virtual colonoscopy has proven to be as accurate as standard endoscopy in identification of polyps.

TEST OF CHOICE
Barium enema or virtual colonoscopy.

BIBLIOGRAPHY
Levin B, Lieberman DA, McFarland B, et al. Screening and surveillance for the early detection of colorectal cancer and adenomatous polyps, 2008: a joint guideline from the American Cancer Society, the US Multi-Society Task Force on Colorectal Cancer, and the American College of Radiology. *Gastroenterology.* 2008 May;134(5):1570-1595. Epub 2008 Feb 8.

Pickhardt PJ, Choi JR, Hwang I, et al. Computed tomographic virtual colonoscopy to screen for colorectal neoplasia in asymptomatic adults. *N Engl J Med.* 2003 Dec 4;349(23):2191-2200. Epub 2003 Dec 1.

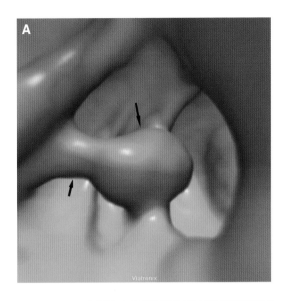

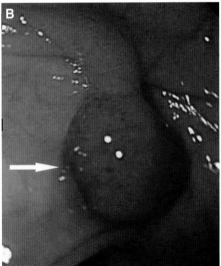

Figure 5-10   (A) Three-dimensional rendering of the internal wall of the colon shows an ovoid polyp on a stalk (arrows). (B) The corresponding image obtained during colonoscopy (arrow).

5-11. Elevated Liver Function Tests with Abdominal Pain

CASE HISTORY
A 50-year-old female presents with elevated liver function tests and abdominal pain.

BACKGROUND
Abnormal liver function and abdominal pain can be due to liver parenchymal disease or biliary obstruction. Worldwide, the most common cause of extrahepatic biliary obstruction is gallstones. The incidence of gallstones increases with age and is much more common in women than in men. Other causes of biliary obstruction include biliary or pancreatic malignancy. However, the most common cause of abnormal liver function in the United States is fatty liver disease. It affects 25%–35% of the population. Fatty liver disease can range from fatty liver alone (steatosis) to fatty liver with inflammation (steatohepatitis) to cirrhosis. Alcohol consumption is one cause but fatty liver can also occur in the absence of alcohol. Nonalcoholic hepatic steatosis (NASH) is associated with obesity, hypertension, and high triglyceride levels.

TEST RATIONALE
It is important to distinguish extrahepatic biliary obstruction from liver disease, as the management of these two conditions is different. Biliary obstruction requires drainage, while hepatic disease is treated medically. Abdominal US is very sensitive and specific (>95%) for identifying biliary ductal dilatation, the hallmark of biliary obstruction (see Fig. 5-11). Conversely, absence of biliary ductal dilatation makes biliary obstruction extremely unlikely, although it does not rule it out entirely. US is therefore the first line imaging study in the patient with pain and abnormal liver function.

If biliary obstruction is found, US can often identify the level and the cause of the obstruction. However, it is less accurate in this regard than MR cholangiopancreatography, or ERCP. These more expensive and invasive tests are usually performed for further evaluation following a positive US.

Advanced fatty liver is readily apparent on US because it results in increased echogenicity of the liver. US is less sensitive to milder degrees of steatosis. MRI is more sensitive than US, but the definitive test is liver biopsy.

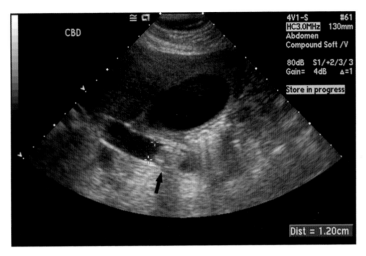

Figure 5-11 Ultrasound shows dilated common bile duct (calipers) obstructed by the bright stone (black arrow).

TEST OF CHOICE
US, followed by MRI, ERCP, or liver biopsy if necessary.

BIBLIOGRAPHY
Foley WD, Quiroz FA. The role of sonography in imaging of the biliary tract. *Ultrasound Q.* 2007 Jun;23(2):123-135.
Laing FC, Jeffrey RB Jr, Wing, et al. Biliary dilatation: defining the level and cause by real-time ultrasound. *Radiology.* 1986 July;160(2):39-42.
Ong JP, Younossi ZM. Approach to the diagnosis and treatment of nonalcoholic fatty liver disease. *Clin Liver Dis.* 2005;9(4):617-34, vi.

5-12. Painless Jaundice

CASE HISTORY
A 60-year-old male with weight loss and jaundice.

BACKGROUND
Pancreatic adenocarcinoma is the commonest pancreatic malignancy. It may present with painless obstructive jaundice or pain radiating to the back. More commonly, patients have vague and nonspecific symptoms such as weight loss. As a result, the disease therefore tends to present in an advanced state and mortality is high. Only 20% of patients are amenable to curative resection at presentation.

TEST RATIONALE
Pancreatic tumors are rarely detectable on clinical examination because of the retroperitoneal location of the organ. Tumor markers are of little utility. Percutaneous sonography is a very accurate method for detecting biliary ductal obstruction, a common sequela of a tumor in the pancreatic head. A negative US is highly specific for excluding biliary obstruction as a cause of jaundice. However, overlying bowel gas and obesity will often limit visualization of the pancreas itself because of the distance of the pancreas from the abdominal wall. Sonography is less sensitive than CT or MR for the detection of pancreatic tumors that do not cause biliary obstruction, particularly tumors located in the pancreatic tail and body. If the US shows biliary obstruction, an MR with Magnetic Resonance Cholangiopancreatography (MRCP) should be performed for further characterization. MRCP has largely replaced ERCP as diagnostic test.

Standard contrast-enhanced multidetector CT or MR are the noninvasive tests of choice for visualizing the entire pancreas, and should be the initial test in patients in nonjaundiced patients with suspected pancreatic cancer (see Figs. 5-12A and 5-12B). CT is generally more readily available than MR. In addition, there are specialized pancreatic CT protocols for cancer staging and for detection of endocrine pancreatic tumors (which have a different clinical presentation).

If a pancreatic mass is found with noninvasive tests, further evaluation can be performed with endoscopic ultrasound (EUS). Biopsy of the pancreatic mass under EUS or CT guidance can provide tissue diagnosis while obstructed bile ducts can be drained during ERCP. PET is useful for cancer staging.

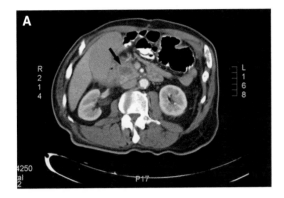

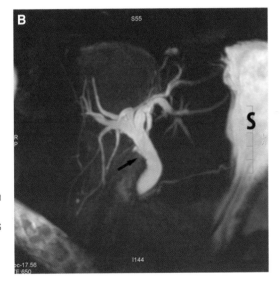

Figure 5-12 (A) Axial contrast-enhanced CT scan shows enlargement of the pancreatic head, consistent with pancreatic cancer (black arrow). (B) The biliary system is bright white on this cholangiogram performed using MRI. There is irregularity of the common bile duct (black arrow) where the pancreatic mass presses on the duct. CT, computed tomography.

TEST OF CHOICE

US if patient is jaundiced, followed by MRCP if the US is positive. Contrast-enhanced CT if the patient is not jaundiced. EUS or ERCP are performed for tissue diagnosis and therapy if cross-sectional imaging is suspicious for a pancreatic neoplasm.

BIBLIOGRAPHY

Foley WD, Quiroz FA. The role of sonography in imaging of the biliary tract. *Ultrasound Q.* 2007;23(2):123-135.

Horton KM, Fishman EK. Adenocarcinoma of the pancreas: CT imaging. *Radiol Clin North Am.* 2002 Dec;40(6):1263-1272.

Michl P, Pauls S, Gress TM. Evidence based diagnosis and staging of pancreatic cancer. *Best Pract Res Clin Gastroenterol.* 2006 Apr;20(2):227-251.

5-13. Abdominal Distention

CASE HISTORY
A 55-year-old male presents with abdominal distension.

BACKGROUND
The majority of patients complaining of bloating and abdominal distension suffer from functional gastrointestinal disorders, such as irritable syndrome, which do not require imaging. However, abdominal distension may indicate ascites, a sign of potentially serious systemic disease. These include portal hypertension due to liver disease, right heart failure, volume overload, and peritoneal malignancy.

IMAGING RATIONALE
US is a quick and accurate method of confirming or ruling out the presence of intraperitoneal free fluid. If the US is normal, no further imaging is necessary. If ascites is found, US with Doppler of the hepatic vasculature is an excellent technique for diagnosing portal hypertension, venous thrombosis, and congestive cardiac failure (see Figs. 5-13A and 5-13B). The finding of varices, porto-systemic collaterals, and splenomegaly on Doppler sonography is strongly suggestive of portal hypertension. Doppler sonography may be followed with contrast-enhanced CT or MR, which are better than US at depicting morphologic changes of cirrhosis in the liver.

TEST OF CHOICE
Abdominal US as the initial study, with Doppler of the hepatic vasculature if the US is abnormal.

BIBLIOGRAPHY

Grant EG, Schiller VL, Millener P. Color Doppler imaging of the hepatic vasculature. *AJR Am J Roentgenol.* 1992 Nov;159(5):943-950.

Zwiebel WJ. Sonographic diagnosis of hepatic vascular disorders. *Semin Ultrasound CT MR.* 1995 Feb;16(1):34-48.

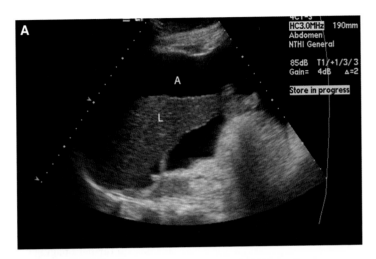

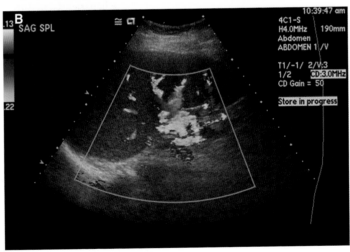

Figure 5-13   (A) Ultrasound examination shows ascites (denoted as A) surrounding a small, nodular cirrhotic liver (denoted as L). (B) Ultrasound image of the liver using Doppler imaging sensitive to blood flow shows reversal of blood flow (blue).

6

DISEASES OF THE GENITOURINARY TRACT

Julia R. Fielding,
Wui K. Chong, and Ellie R. Lee

6-1. Incidental Renal Mass

CASE HISTORY
A 50-year-old male with abnormal abdominal physical examination, presents with a solid mass identified on recent ultrasound (US).

BACKGROUND
The majority of renal tumors are incidentally detected on computed tomography (CT) or US during evaluation for other diseases or unrelated symptoms. Forty percent of adults over 40 years of age will have a renal lesion. The vast majority of these lesions will be benign cysts, and require no follow-up. Solid masses are considered malignant until proven otherwise. In adults, the most common type of kidney cancer is renal cell carcinoma, which accounts for 90%–95% of renal neoplasms and for approximately 3% of adult malignancies. This most commonly occurs in men in the fourth to sixth decades of life. Hematuria is uncommon. The majority of patients with renal cell carcinoma are asymptomatic. Renal cell carcinoma develops in approximately 30%–40% of patients with Von Hippel–Lindau disease.

TEST RATIONALE
Contrast-enhanced CT scanning is the imaging procedure of choice for diagnosis and staging renal cell carcinoma. CT imaging can help differentiate cystic masses from solid masses. Renal cell carcinoma demonstrates significant contrast enhancement (see Fig. 6-1). CT imaging can provide information about lymph nodes, renal vein, and inferior vena cava involvement for staging. At the time of diagnosis, 30% of renal cell carcinoma has spread to the ipsilateral renal vein and 5%–10% has continued into the inferior vena cava. If further evaluation is needed, magnetic resonance imaging (MRI) angiography is the next imaging study for detecting inferior cava tumor thrombus involvement. Also, CT can assess for distant metastatic lesions, typically occurring in the lungs, liver, and adrenal glands. Early detection and accurate staging is important in surgical management and prognosis. Renal lesions <3 cm in size can be appropriately treated with conservative nephron-sparing surgery, either partial nephrectomy or tumor enucleation and, in some cases, radiofrequency ablation. Renal lesions >3 cm are usually treated with radical nephrectomy.

TEST OF CHOICE
CT scan.
Coutrast-enhanced

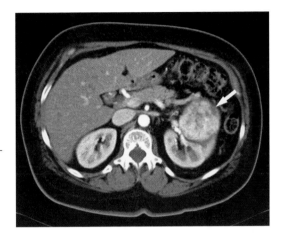

Figure 6-1 Renal cell carcinoma. Axial contrast-enhanced CT image of the left kidney. There is a large heterogeneously enhancing mass in the mid left kidney (arrow).

BIBLIOGRAPHY

Catalano C, Fraioli F, Laghi A, et al. High resolution multidetector CT in the preoperative evaluation of patients with renal cell carcinoma. *AJR*. 2003 (May);180(5):1271-1277.

Reznek R. CT/MRI in staging renal cell carcinoma. *Cancer Imaging.* 2004 Feb;4:S25-S32.

6-2. Painful Testicle

CASE HISTORY
A 5-year-old male presents with right scrotal pain.

BACKGROUND
Testicular torsion occurs when there is twisting of the spermatic cord, which cuts off the blood supply to the testicle and the surrounding structures within the scrotum causing testicular ischemia. The condition is more common during infancy (first year of life) and adolescence (puberty), 10–20 years old, but can happen at any age. Some men may be predisposed to testicular torsion as a result of inadequate connective tissue within the scrotum. Risk factors are trauma and strenuous physical activity. Clinical presentation includes sudden onset of pain, nausea and vomiting, low-grade fever, swollen and tender hemiscrotum, and absent cremasteric reflex. Differential diagnosis includes epididymo-orchitis (infection or inflammation), testicular cancer, and trauma.

If the condition is diagnosed quickly and corrected immediately, the testicle may be salvaged. If surgery is performed within 6 hours, most testicles can be saved. After 6 hours of torsion (impaired blood flow), the testicle is at risk for dying and the likelihood that the testicle will need to be removed increases. However, even with less than 6 hours of torsion, the testicle may lose its ability to function. This is an emergency and surgery should be performed as soon as possible after symptoms begin. The testicle on the other (nonaffected) side is at risk of testicular torsion and usually also anchored during surgery as a preventive measure.

TEST RATIONALE
Many causes of acute scrotal pain, including testicular torsion, epididymo-orchitis, and intratesticular tumor have similar clinical presentation. Ultrasonography is the imaging modality of choice for examination of the scrotum. Color and power Doppler US can be used to determine testicular perfusion. In testicular torsion, the blood supply to the testicles and surrounding tissues is cut off. Therefore, color Doppler US can demonstrate the absence of blood flow to the testicle (see Figs. 6-2A and 6-2B). In testicular torsion, first obstruction of the venous flow occurs, followed by obstruction of the arterial flow and subsequently testicular ischemia. This can distinguish it from another common cause of testicular pain, epididymitis, where increased blood flow is seen. Also, testicular masses can be excluded.

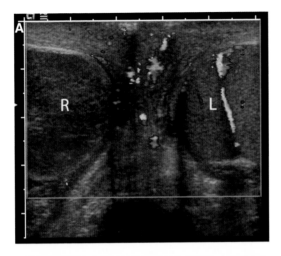

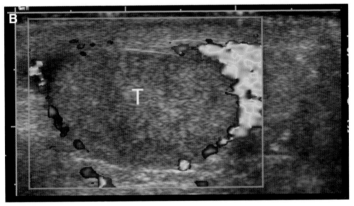

Figure 6-2   (A) Right testicular torsion. Color Doppler ultrasound image of the right (R) and left (L) testicles. Color blood flow (red and blue) is identified in the left testicle indicating normal blood flow. Also, color blood flow is identified in the scrotal tissues between the testicles. No color blood flow is identified in the right testicle. The right testicle is hypoechoic (darker) as compared to the normal left testicle indicating edema. (B) Right testicular torsion. Color Doppler ultrasound image of the right testicle. The right testicle (T) demonstrates heterogeneous echotexture and no intratesticular blood flow, indicating testicular ischemia. There is color blood flow in the scrotal tissue surrounding the right testicle representing increased paratesticular flow related to hyperemia.

TEST OF CHOICE
Testicular US.

BIBLIOGRAPHY
Dogra V, Bhatt S. Acute painful scrotum. *Radiol Clin North Am.* 2004 Mar;42(2):349-363.
Dogra VS, Gottlieb RH, Oka M, Rubens DJ. Sonography of the scrotum. *Radiology.* 2003 Apr;227(1):18-36. Epub 2003 Feb 28.

6-3. Painful Hematuria

CASE HISTORY
A 48-year-old male presents with left flank pain and hematuria.

BACKGROUND
Renal calculi are a common cause for blood in the urine and pain in the abdomen, flank, or groin. This occurs in 1 in 20 people. Development of the stones is related to decreased urine volume or increased excretion of stone-forming components such as calcium, oxalate, urate, cystine, xanthine, and phosphate. The most common causes for painful hematuria are renal calculus, pyelonephritis/urinary tract infection, trauma, and neoplasms with resultant passage of clots. Common presenting symptoms include acute flank pain, radiating colicky pain, or dysuria with hematuria.

TEST RATIONALE
Almost all urinary calculi are radiodense and can be detected on nonenhanced CT. The exception is radiolucent crystal depositions in the urinary tract related to protease inhibitor therapy for human immunovirus (HIV), indinavir (Crixivan; Merck, Rahway, NJ). Previously other imaging modalities, such as conventional radiographs, intravenous pyelogram, and US have been performed. However, nonenhanced CT has a higher sensitivity (95%–98%) for the detection of ureteral calculi and other clinically relevant information, including acute obstruction, position, and accurate size of calculus for treatment planning (see Figs. 6-3A and 6-3B). Small less than 5 mm calculi will likely pass spontaneously (90%) and usually treated with hydration and analgesics. Larger calculi greater than 8 mm will rarely pass and may require surgical intervention. Also, nonenhanced CT may be helpful in detecting other diagnoses for the patient's pain, such as appendicitis, diverticulitis, pancreatitis, tubo-ovarian abscess, malignancy, and ruptured aortic aneurysm.

TEST OF CHOICE
Nonenhanced CT.

BIBLIOGRAPHY
Boulay I, Holtz P, Foley WD, et al. Ureteral calculi: diagnostic efficacy of helical CT and implications for treatment of patients. *AJR.* 1999 June;172(6):1485-1490.
Sheafor DH, Hertzberg BS, Freed KS, et al. Nonenhanced helical CT and US in the emergency evaluation of patients with renal colic: prospective comparison. *Radiology.* 2000 Dec;217(3):792-797.

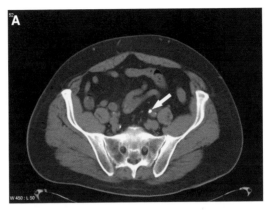

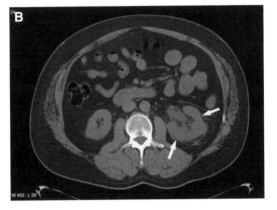

Figure 6-3 (A) Nonenhanced transaxial CT image of the pelvis demonstrates a 6 mm calculus in the left mid ureter (arrow). Surrounding rim of soft tissue and periureteral stranding is identified.
(B) Nonenhanced transaxial CT image demonstrates an enlarged left kidney with moderate hydronephrosis and perinephric stranding representing acute obstruction (arrows). CT, computed tomography.

6-4. Painless Vaginal Bleeding

CASE HISTORY
A 77-year-old postmenopausal female presents with vaginal bleeding.

BACKGROUND
Postmenopausal vaginal bleeding is defined as spontaneous vaginal bleeding that occurs more than 1 year after the date of the last menstrual period and not related to bleeding associated with hormone-replacement therapy. Postmenopausal vaginal bleeding is the most common presenting symptom of endometrial cancer. Endometrial cancer occurs in approximately 10% of women with postmenopausal bleeding. It is the most common gynecologic malignancy and the fourth most common cancer in U.S. women, affecting 1 in 50. It commonly occurs in women over 50 years old. In endometrial cancer, the endometrium is diffusely thickened, irregular, and echogenic. Endometrial cancer less commonly appears as a broad-based polypoid endometrial mass. Endometrial cancer is usually preceded by endometrial hyperplasia. Adenocarcinoma accounts for >80% of endometrial cancers. Major risk factors are obesity, diabetes, and hypertension. Other risk factors include unopposed estrogen, tamoxifen use for greater than 5 years, previous pelvic radiation therapy, and a personal or family history of breast or ovarian cancer.

Other causes of postmenopausal vaginal bleeding include endometrial atrophy (59%), endometrial polyp (12%), endometrial hyperplasia (10%), hormonal effect (7%), cervical cancer (2%), and fibroids.

TEST RATIONALE
A 2000 Consensus Conference Statement from the Society of Radiologists in Ultrasound recommended that either transvaginal US or endometrial biopsy could be used safely and effectively in the initial evaluation of patients with postmenopausal bleeding (see Figs. 6-4A and 6-4B). Using an endometrial thickness measurement of >5 mm as abnormal, they concluded that the sensitivities of transvaginal US and endometrial biopsy are comparable when sufficient tissue is obtained with endometrial biopsy. The sensitivity for detecting endometrial carcinoma approaches 95% when an endometrial thickness threshold 5 mm is used. Transvaginal US is tolerated better and has a higher rate (>95%) of diagnostic results. Also, transvaginal US can also help identify other causes of postmenopausal bleeding, such as polyps, fibroids, or atypical hyperplasia. Saline infused sonohysterography or hysteroscopy can be performed next when a focal abnormality is

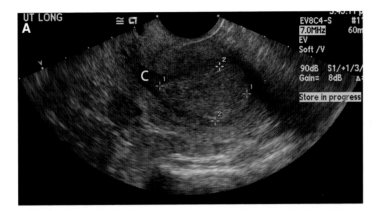

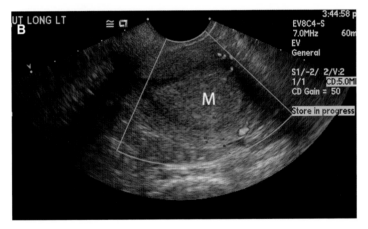

Figure 6-4   (A) Endometrial cancer. Endovaginal ultrasound image of the uterus. Large heterogeneous mass (between 1 and 2 calipers) is identified within the endometrium (outlined in black). The uterus is outlined by arrows. The cervix (c) is partially visualized. (B) Endometrial cancer. Endovaginal ultrasound image of the uterus. The endometrial mass demonstrates blood flow (blue and red).

suspected on transvaginal US. If a diffuse abnormality is found, a patient can proceed to endometrial biopsy and D & C. All patients with postmenopausal bleeding require close follow-up.

TEST OF CHOICE
Transvaginal US.

BIBLIOGRAPHY
Goldstein RB, Bree RL, Benacerraf BR et al. Evaluation of the woman with postmenopausal bleeding society of radiologists in ultrasound-sponsored consensus conference statement. *J Ultrasound Med*. 2001 Oct;20(10):1025-1036.
Smith-Bindman R, Kerlikowski K, Felstein Va, et al. Endovaginal ultrasound to exclude endometrial cancer and other endometrial abnormalities. *JAMA*. 1998 Nov;280(17):1510-1517.

6-5. Painful Adnexal Mass

CASE HISTORY
A 22-year-old female presents with bilateral pelvic pain and fever.

BACKGROUND
Pelvic inflammatory disease (PID) is an infection of the female upper genital tract, which results from an ascending infection of the vagina or cervix that progresses to endometritis followed by salpingitis and salpingo-oophoritis. Cervical motion tenderness combined with organisms identified in vaginal fluid are clinical findings pathognomonic for PID. Adhesions may develop within the fallopian tubes, causing tubal obstruction, dilation, and infection (pyosalpinx). Inadequately treated PID can lead to infection of the ovary with resultant unilateral or bilateral tubo-ovarian abscesses or rupture, which can result in life-threatening generalized peritonitis. The peak incidence rate is in women aged 20–24 years. The incidence of tubo-ovarian abscess has increased as a result of increase in sexually transmitted diseases. Patients with tubo-ovarian abscess most commonly present with lower abdominal pain and an adnexal mass. Fever and leukocytosis may be present. Tubo-ovarian abscess is polymicrobial with a prevalence of anaerobic organism, such as *Chlamydia trachomatis* or *Neisseria gonorrhea*. Other conditions that can mimic pelvic abscess/tubo-ovarian abscess include necrotic pelvic neoplasm, hematoma, hemorrhagic physiologic cyst, ectopic pregnancy, and endometrioma.

TEST RATIONALE
Endovaginal US provides detailed examination of the uterus and adnexa, including the fallopian tubes and ovaries. US is readily available and noninvasive with no radiation exposure. Also, it can be performed at the patient's bedside. Hydrosalpinx or pyosalpinx is a dilated tube, which may contain dark fluid and debris. Tubo-ovarian abscesses are usually solid and cystic masses that involve the ovary with thickened walls and central fluid (see Figs. 6-5A and 6-5B). Significant blood flow is identified in most cases of tubo-ovarian abscesses with color Doppler US. Most cases of PID improve with an antibiotic regimen. Significant pelvic abscesses may need to be drained percutaneously or surgically.

TEST OF CHOICE
Pelvic US.

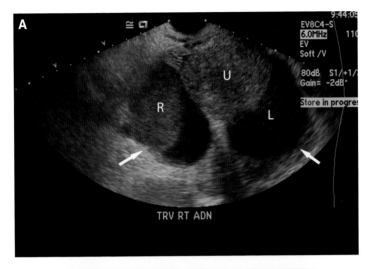

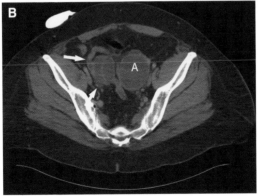

Figure 6-5   (A) Transvaginal ultrasound of the pelvis. Right (R) and left (L) large complex ovarian masses compatible with tubo-ovarian abscesses (arrows). Uterus (U). (B) Nonenhanced transaxial CT image of the pelvis. Complex cystic lesion in the left adnexa, compatible with tubo-ovarian abscess (denoted as A). Complex cystic lesion in the right adnexa with a tubular appearance, compatible with hydrosalpinx/pyosalpinx (arrows).

BIBLIOGRAPHY

Jeong WK, Kim Y, Song S. Tubo-ovarian abscess: CT and pathologic correlation. *Clinical Imaging*. 2007 Nov-Dec;31(6):414-418.

Wilbur AC, Aizenstein RI, Napp TE. CT findings in tuboovarian abscess. *AJR*. 1992 Mar;158(3):575-579.

6-6. Painful Pelvic Mass

CASE HISTORY
A 32-year-old female presents with chronic pelvic pain.

BACKGROUND
There are numerous causes for pelvic pain. Beyond the gynecologic organs, pathology of the muscles, small and large bowel, and vascular system should be considered. The majority of these can be eliminated using a focused history and physical examination. In many cases, bowel adhesions, often due to endometriosis, are the likely source of pain. Endometriosis and its complications are usually diagnosed and treated using laparoscopy. Preoperative imaging is performed to search for endometriomas.

TEST RATIONALE
Endometriomas are contained collections of endometrial glandular tissue located beyond the endometrium. They are most commonly located adjacent to the ovary and fallopian tubes, along the posterior wall of the uterus, within the cul de sac and adjacent to the rectum. The customary US appearance of an adnexal endometrioma is that of a uniformly echogenic mass, round to ovoid in shape with through transmission of the sound wave, indicating that it contains fluid (see Figs. 6-6A and 6-6B). This is sometimes referred to as a chocolate cyst. If the adnexal mass cannot be clearly identified as an endometrioma, or if multiple sites of disease are suspected, MRI can be performed before laparoscopy.

TEST OF CHOICE
Transvaginal US.

BIBLIOGRAPHY
Gougoutas CA, Siegelman ES, Hunt J, et al. Pelvic endometriosis, various manifestations and MR imaging findings, *AJR*. 2000 Aug;(2);175:353-358.

Jeong YY, Outwater EK, Hang HK. Imaging evaluation of ovarian masses. *Radiographics*. 2000 Sept-Oct;20(5):1445-1470.

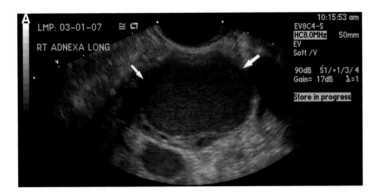

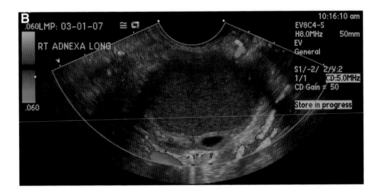

Figure 6-6 (A) Ultrasound image of a pelvic mass that contains debris (arrows). (B) The lack of color inside the mass indicated that it does not have a vascular supply and is therefore not a neoplasm.

6-7. Infertility

CASE HISTORY
A 36-year-old female presents with inability to conceive over the last year.

BACKGROUND
The most common cause of infertility in women over the age of 35 is primary ovarian failure. However, the anatomy of the uterus and fallopian tubes must be assessed to identify any obstacle to fertilization of the ovum or implantation of the conceptus. Common abnormalities include fibroids and tubal occlusion. Most tubal disease is secondary to PID. Sequelae of infection include obstruction and dilation of the distal fallopian tube (hydrosalpinx). Adhesions may also be seen surrounding the ovary. Uncommonly, congenital uterine anomalies such as a duplication or agenesis are present.

TEST RATIONALE
Despite the use of ionizing radiation, the single best test for assessing tubal patency is the hysterosalpingogram (HSG). In the test, a catheter is introduced through the cervix and a small volume of iodine-based contrast agent injected into the uterus and fallopian tubes. This test requires only a few minutes to complete, is readily available, and accurate for identification of fallopian tube disease. Uterine abnormalities can also be identified and further assessed using hysteroscopy, three-dimensional US or in some cases MRI.

TEST OF CHOICE
Hysterosalpingogram.

BIBLIOGRAPHY
Thurmond AS. Imaging of female infertility. *Radiol Clin North Am.* 2002;41:757-767.

6-8. Prostate Cancer

CASE HISTORY
A 62-year-old man presents with an enlarged prostate gland and a prostate specific antigen (PSA) level of 40 mg/dl.

BACKGROUND
The risk factors for prostate cancer include increased age, a high fat diet, and a family history of breast or prostate cancer. By age 75, nearly 75% of men will have cancerous cells within the prostate. Fortunately, most of these cancers will not progress to active disease. An abnormal digital rectal examination and elevated PSA level, usually defined as >4 ng/ml, detect the majority of early-curable prostate cancer. PSA level does not correlate with the tumor aggressiveness, although it serves as an accurate marker for progression of disease.

TEST RATIONALE
Transrectal ultrasonography (TRUS) is used to guide a core biopsy needle into the prostate. Twelve samples are removed, 10 from the periphery and 2 from the central portion of the gland. The systematic sampling is required because TRUS cannot accurately localize the disease within the gland. The samples are then graded using the Gleason criteria, which sum the grade of the most aggressive histologic sample with that of the most prevalent. Those patients with a Gleason sum of <7 and a PSA <10 mg/ml are considered to have curable disease and go directly to therapy.

If the patient is felt to be at high risk for advanced disease (PSA >10 ng/ml, Gleason score >7) imaging tests that detect systemic spread should be considered. Using a standard Tc99m diphosphonate bone scan, approximately 10% of patients with PSA >10 ng/ml will have bony metastases at presentation. A CT scan can evaluate whether the tumor has extended into the bladder and presence or absence of lymphadenopathy, and is routinely ordered when PSA exceeds 20 mg/ml (see Figs. 6-8A and 6-8B). CT is not a reliable test for evaluation of prostate capsule penetration or local extension of disease.

TEST OF CHOICE
TRUS guided biopsy, bone scan, CT scan.

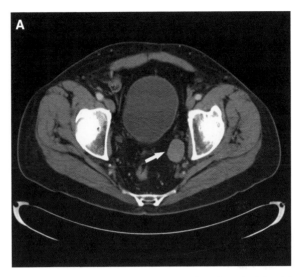

Figure 6-8 (A) Axial CT scan shows an enlarged lymph node on the left pelvic sidewall (arrow). (B) Axial CT more inferiorly shows recurrent disease in the prostate bed (arrow). Rectum is labeled R and bladder B. CT, computed tomography.

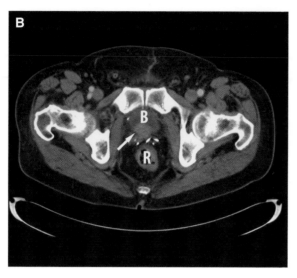

Figure 6-8   Continued.

BIBLIOGRAPHY

Albertsen PC, Hanley JA, Harlan LC, et al. The positive yield of imaging studies in the evaluation of men with newly diagnosed prostate cancer: a population based analysis. *J Urol.* 2000 Apr;163(4):1138-1143.

Chang, SS. Amin, MB. Utilizing the tumor-node-metastasis staging for prostate cancer: the sixth edition, 2002. *CA Cancer J Clin.* 2008 Jan-Feb;58(1):54-59, Epub 2007 Dec 20.

6-9. Transitional Cell Carcinoma

CASE HISTORY
A 65-year-old male presents with painless hematuria.

BACKGROUND
The most common causes of painless hematuria are stones, prostate enlargement (in a male), and urinary tract infections (in a female). However, at least 10% of transitional cell carcinomas (TCC) arising from the urothelial lining present with hematuria. Risk factors include age >65 years, smoking history, and male gender.

TEST RATIONALE
Since 90% of TCC occurs in the bladder, all patients undergo cystoscopy. Direct visualization allows for detection and biopsy. Radiologic tests are employed to assess the upper tracts for synchronous tumors. The test of choice in the high-risk patient is the CT urogram (see Figs. 6-9A and 6-9B). In this test contrast-enhanced CT images are reformatted in the coronal plane. Tumors can be identified and staged using a single examination. If this test is not available or in low-risk patients, such as young active men or women, a standard intravenous urogram (IVU) can be used. This test will identify lesions arising from the renal pelvis or ureter with little radiation exposure. The IVU will not identify renal cell carcinoma, which is an unusual source of hematuria, or evidence of metastatic disease. Patients with TCC are at risk for metachronous tumors and usually undergo periodic screening for several years following detection and treatment of the primary tumor.

TEST OF CHOICE
CT urogram.

BIBLIOGRAPHY
Canfield SE, Dinney CPN, Droller MJ. Surveillance and management of recurrence for upper tract transitional cell carcinoma. *Urol Clin N Am.* 2003 Nov;30(4):791-802.
Webb JA. Imaging in hematuria. *Clin Radiol.* 1997Mar;52(3):167-171.

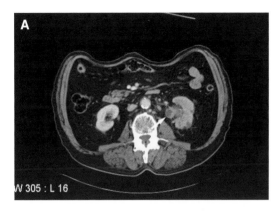

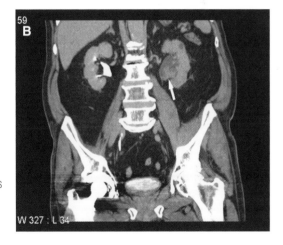

Figure 6-9 (A) Axial CT shows a mass in the left renal pelvis (arrow). (B) Coronal CT shows delayed excretion on the left secondary to the mass (arrow). CT, computed tomography.

6-10. Urethral Trauma

CASE HISTORY
A 19-year-old male presents with urethral bleeding after being struck by a car.

BACKGROUND
Urethral bleeding is concerning for partial or complete urethral rupture. Bladder injury or intraperitoneal rupture are also concerning following trauma, although these typically don't present with urethral bleeding. Classic signs for urethral rupture include blood at the urethral meatus and a full bladder with the inability to void. Other signs include a high riding prostate upon rectal examination, hematuria (91%–100% urethral injuries present with hematuria) and extravasation of blood in the perineum. Urethral injuries are classified as either posterior or anterior. Posterior urethral injuries tend to occur from traumas causing rapid decelerations, such as motor vehicle accidents and major falls. They are often associated with pelvic fractures and almost always require surgical intervention, either immediate or delayed. Anterior urethral injury occurs from blunt trauma to the perineum, usually from straddle injuries or traumatic catheter insertion. These injuries may need immediate intervention, but many can be observed. Anterior injuries often present with urethral stricture many years later.

TEST RATIONALE
In a trauma case, the patient must be stabilized before tending to a possible urethral rupture. Often a trauma patient will undergo a CT scan pelvis as part of the trauma series. These are typically not beneficial in evaluating the urethra itself, but may indicate a more serious pelvic fracture, which should be further stabilized before tending to the urethra. All suspected urethral ruptures or bladder injuries require a retrograde urethrogram (RUG) before a catheter can be inserted. The test will show whether a rupture is present and will qualify whether the injury is complete or partial, or whether the urethra is stretched or compressed. The RUG is ideally performed under fluoroscopy so extravasation of contrast can be detected in real-time. However, if fluoroscopy is unavailable the test should not be delayed.

It was once common practice to use catheter insertion as a diagnostic tool to rule out urethral rupture with the assumption that an injured urethra would prevent catheter advancement. This has become universally condemned, as it frequently leads to further damage to partial urethral tears and may contaminate a sterile hematoma. If, however, a catheter is inserted before a RUG, it should remain in place.

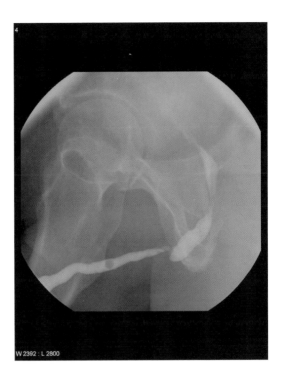

Figure 6-10 The male urethra is opacified. The abrupt change in caliber indicated a healed site of trauma.

In recent years, the utilization of MR and US to diagnose urethral injuries has increased. In the trauma setting, RUG remains the gold-standard as it quickly and clearly shows damage to the urethra itself (see Fig. 6-10). MR and US are often useful as presurgical tests as they show the condition of the soft tissue surrounding the urethra and provide more information to the reconstructing urologist. However, they should not be considered first-line tests.

TEST OF CHOICE
Retrograde urethrogram (RUG).

BIBLIOGRAPHY
Koraitim MM. Pelvic fracture urethral injuries: the unresolved controversy. *J Urol.* 1999 May;161(5):1433-1441.
Pavlica P, Barozzi L, Menchi I. Imaging of male urethra. *Eur Radiol.* 2003 July;13(7):1583-1596. Epub 2002 Dec 19.

6-11. Painless Renal Failure or Elevation in Serum Creatinine

CASE HISTORY

A 70-year-old presents with elevation in serum creatinine and no other symptoms.

BACKGROUND

Renal failure can be classified as (a) prerenal, due to volume depletion (b) renal disease, due to nephron injury, and (c) postrenal, due to urinary tract obstruction. Most cases of painless renal failure are due to renal or prerenal causes. As a rule, an obstruction would have to be bilateral to cause failure of renal function. The most common causes of obstructive renal failure are bladder outlet obstruction due to prostatic enlargement in men or pelvic tumor in women. Obstruction is rarely the cause of painless renal failure in the absence of a distended bladder or a pelvic mass.

TEST RATIONALE

US can be helpful for evaluation of parenchymal renal disease to a limited degree (see Fig. 6-11). The kidneys may appear normal but it is more usual to see increased cortical echogenicity, which is a nonspecific indicator of parenchymal renal disease. Polycystic renal disease has a characteristic sonographic appearance. The finding of small kidneys and cortical thinning indicates chronic renal insufficiency.

The sonographic finding of hydronephrosis is highly accurate for diagnosis and exclusion of urinary tract obstruction. If hydronephrosis is seen and the cause is not identified, the patient should proceed to CT or MR. Intravenous-contrast agents should not be used if serum creatinine is above 2.0.

TEST OF CHOICE

As painless renal failure is uncommonly due to obstruction, no imaging test is indicated in many cases, particularly where there is no clinical evidence of urinary retention or pelvic mass. If obstruction is suspected, US should be the initial test of choice, followed by CT or MR if necessary.

BIBLIOGRAPHY

Keyserling HF, Fielding JR, Mittelstaedt CA. Renal sonography in the intensive care unit: when is it necessary? *J Ultrasound Med.* 2002 May;21(5):517-520.

Khati NJ, Hill MC, Kimmel PL. The role of ultrasound in renal insufficiency: the essentials. *Ultrasound Quarterly.* 2005 Dec;21(4):227-244.

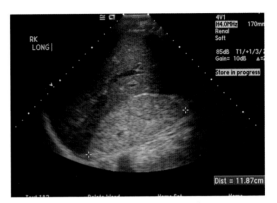

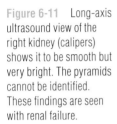

Figure 6-11 Long-axis ultrasound view of the right kidney (calipers) shows it to be smooth but very bright. The pyramids cannot be identified. These findings are seen with renal failure.

6-12. Ectopic Pregnancy

CASE HISTORY
Pelvic pain and bleeding in 7-week pregnant patient.

BACKGROUND
Ectopic pregnancy is caused by implantation of the gestational sac outside the uterus, usually in the fallopian tube. Rupture of an ectopic pregnancy is a potentially lethal complication. The classic clinical triad of pain, vaginal bleeding, and a palpable adnexal mass, is only found in 45% of patients with ectopic pregnancy. Other causes of pain and bleeding include spontaneous abortion.

TEST RATIONALE
US is the imaging study of choice in first trimester of pregnancy. The gestational age can be determined by the β HCG level. An intrauterine gestational sac should be visible with a transvaginal sonography above a threshold β HCG level of 2,000 mIU/ml (WHO International Reference Preparation), which corresponds to 5-week gestation. Identification of an intrauterine gestational sac excludes an ectopic pregnancy, (except in the rare instance of a coexisting ectopic and intrauterine twin pregnancy). Absence of a sac raises the possibility of an ectopic pregnancy but can also be found in spontaneous abortion. Identification of an ectopic gestational sac in the adnexa is specific for ectopic pregnancy (see Fig. 6-12). US can also detect intraperitoneal free fluid, which in the setting of an ectopic pregnancy is indicative of rupture.

TEST OF CHOICE
Transvaginal US, correlated with serum β HCG.

BIBLIOGRAPHY
Brown DL, Doubilet PM. Transvaginal sonography for diagnosing ectopic pregnancy: positivity criteria and performance characteristics. *J Ultrasound Med.* 1994 Apr; (4);13:259-266.

Daya S, Woods S, Ward S, et al. Transvaginal ultrasound scanning in early pregnancy and correlation with human chorionic gonadotropin levels. *J Clin Ultrasound.* 1991 Mar-Apr;19 (3):139-142.

Schwartz RO, Di Pietro DL. Beta HCG as a diagnostic aid for suspected ectopic pregnancy. *Obstet Gynecol.* 1980 Aug;56(2):197-203.

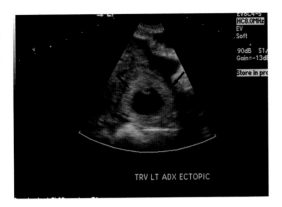

Figure 6-12 Ultrasound examination of the left aspect of the pelvis shows a ring-shaped structure (arrows) with black fluid within it. If the pregnancy test is positive and there is no intrauterine pregnancy seen this finding is highly suspicious for an ectopic pregnancy within a fallopian tube.

6-13. Abdominal Pain and Pregnancy

CASE HISTORY
A 25-year-old pregnant female presents with abdominal pain.

BACKGROUND
Imaging of the abdomen and pelvis in pregnancy is constrained by the need to minimize fetal exposure to radiation. Potentially harmful radiation effects of vary depending on the fetal stage of development and the magnitude of the dose and this has to be weighed against the state of the mother's health. Where possible, radiation should be avoided particularly in the first and the second trimester.

IMAGING RATIONALE
US and MRI do not use ionizing radiation and should be used in place of CT or radiography whenever possible. US has no adverse effects on the fetus and is the modality of choice if obstetric, ovarian, or gall bladder pathology is suspected. US is also of value if appendicitis or urinary tract obstruction is suspected particularly in the first trimester of pregnancy (see Fig. 6-13). However, US is less helpful in urinary obstruction than in non-pregnant patients because of physiologic nonobstructive hydronephrosis of pregnancy, which can be difficult to differentiate from obstruction.

There have been no adverse effects described with MRI in pregnancy. Nevertheless, MRI should be avoided in the first trimester during organogenesis, and MR-contrast agents are not used, because their effects on the fetus are not clear. MR provides a global view of the entire abdomen and pelvis and is the test of choice if bowel, pancreatic, or retroperitoneal pathology is suspected. At many institutions, MRI is now the primary test used to diagnose appendicitis in the pregnant patient.

CT is performed when an intravenous-contrasted study is required, such as trauma or evaluation for vascular or ischemic pathology.

TEST OF CHOICE
US and/or MRI; CT when there is no alternative.

BIBLIOGRAPHY
Fielding JR, Chin BM. Magnetic resonance imaging of abdominal pain during pregnancy. *Top Magn Reson Imaging*. 2006 Dec;17(6):409-416.

Figure 6-13 Mild hydronephrosis is commonly seen during pregnancy as the uterus presses on the ureter. Ultrasound image shows an obstructed left kidney. The arrows point to dilated calyces filled with urine. This may be due to a distal obstructing stone or mass.

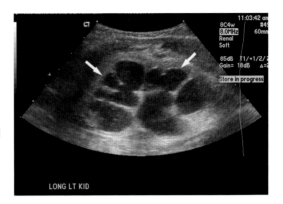

7

DISEASES OF THE MUSCULOSKELETAL SYSTEM

Nancy M. Major and
Taymon Domzalski

7-1. Ankle Pain

CASE HISTORY
A 25-year-old female with ankle inversion injury was brought in to the emergency room; the ankle is too painful for the patient to bear weight.

BACKGROUND
Ankle sprain is a very common injury. It has been estimated that approximately 25,000 children and adults experience an ankle injury every day, in varying degrees of severity. Sprains constitute 85% of all ankle injuries and 85% of ankle sprains are due to inversion injury. It is important to correctly diagnose these injuries because up to 40% of patients with untreated or misdiagnosed ankle injuries develop chronic symptoms.

TEST RATIONALE
The most important test for ankle sprains is a good clinical examination. Most patients with ankle sprains have pain, but it is up to the clinician to determine the severity of the injury. The Ottawa ankle rules are currently the best guidelines to follow in helping the physician decide if the injury is severe enough to warrant conventional radiographs of the foot/ankle. Use of the rules has led to a decrease in ankle radiography, waiting times, and costs without an increased rate of missed fractures. According to the Ottawa ankle rules, conventional radiographs are necessary only if there is pain in the malleolar or midfoot area (see Fig. 7-1), and any one of the following:

1. Tenderness along the distal 6 cm of the posterior edge of the fibula or tip of the lateral malleolus
2. Tenderness along the distal 6 cm of the posterior edge of the tibia or tip of the medial malleolus
3. Tenderness at the navicular bone
4. Tenderness at the base of the fifth metatarsal
5. An inability to bear weight for four steps. If the patient is able to bear weight and ambulate on the affected ankle, without severe pain, they are unlikely to have a fracture or torn tendon/ligament. These patients need no further testing.

Pregnant women, children, and obtunded patients (that is, head injury or intoxication) should not be evaluated utilizing these guidelines.

TEST OF CHOICE
If the patient cannot ambulate or bear weight on affected ankle, begin radiographic evaluation with conventional radiographs of the ankle looking for

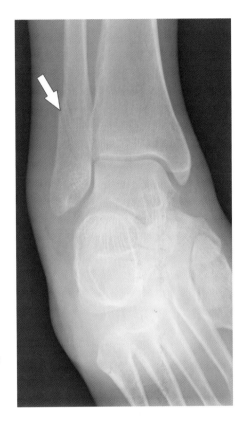

Figure 7-1   Patient is status post-ankle inversion injury. While the anterior posterior view did not show the fracture this oblique view of the joint (mortise view) shows a spiral fracture of the distal fibula (arrow).

fractures. If no fractures are seen and the patient continues to have severe pain out of proportion to ligament injury, a magnetic resonance imaging (MRI) of the ankle is indicated to evaluate the soft tissues and occult fracture.

BIBLIOGRAPHY

Rimando MP. "Ankle Sprain." eMedicine. April 10, 2008 http://www.emedicine.com/pmr/TOPIC11.HTM

Stiell I, Wells G, Laupacis A, et al. Multicentre trial to introduce the Ottawa ankle rules for use of radiography in acute ankle injuries. Multicentre Ankle Rule Study Group. *BMJ*. 1995 Sep 2;311(7005):594-597.

7-2. Osteomyelitis

CASE HISTORY
A 62-year-old diabetic female complains to her doctor of a red, hot, swollen foot.

BACKGROUND
There are several routes of infection into the bone: direct implantation from a penetrating wound, contiguous spread from soft tissue or cellulitis, and hematogenous spread. Osteomyelitis has a variable appearance on conventional radiographs. That is, it may or may not be expansile, may or may not have a well-defined margin, or be associated with periosteal reaction.

TEST RATIONALE
Radionuclide bone scan imaging is more sensitive than conventional radiography, but it is not specific for osteomyelitis. It can become positive hours to days after the onset of symptoms. A bone scan is helpful to evaluate additional sites of involvement, and it can support the diagnosis, but it is not specific for osteomyelitis when positive. MRI, on the other hand, is very sensitive, especially when associated fluid collections or abscesses are identified. There are, however, many causes of abnormal bone marrow signal on MRI. Osteomyelitis is just one of those causes. If cortical destruction is seen with MRI, or if a fluid collection is noted within the bone, these findings would be virtually diagnostic of osteomyelitis (see Figs. 7-2A and 7-2B). MRI is especially helpful when the bone marrow signal is normal. If the marrow is normal, there is NO osteomyelitis.

TEST OF CHOICE
If a soft tissue abscess or sinus tract is present, MRI is the test of choice. If no obvious cause of the pain is present use a 3-phase bone scan as a localizer to narrow the field of view, utilizing MRI for definitive diagnosis.

BIBLIOGRAPHY
King, RW. "Osteomyelitis." eMedicine. May 12, 2008. Available at http://www.emedicine.com/emerg/topic349.HTM
Major NM. *A Practical Approach to Radiology*. Philadelphia, PA: W.B. Saunders, 2006:115-119.

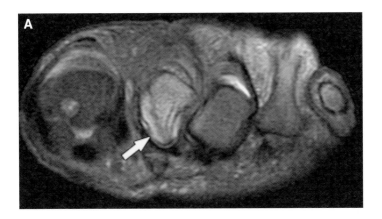

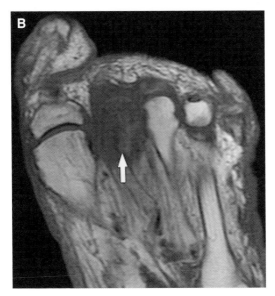

Figure 7-2   Osteomyeitis. (A) Short axis T2 weighted image through the second meta-tarsal head. Abnormal bone marrow edema is noted in the head of the second metatarsal (arrow). (B) Long axis T1 weighted image demonstrates bone destruction (loss of cortex) (arrow). Bone destruction is diagnostic of osteomyelitis.

7-3. Rheumatoid Arthritis

CASE HISTORY
A 53-year-old complains of worsening knee pain. The patient has prior plain films consistent with rheumatoid arthritis.

BACKGROUND
Rheumatoid arthritis is an inflammatory arthritis that is symmetric in distribution and is characterized by erosions and osteoporosis. In the hands, the arthritis typically affects the wrist before the fingers. However, it can affect any synovial joint in the body. Soft tissue swelling is a prominent feature and often affects the region of the ulnar styloid process. Joint-space narrowing that occurs with rheumatoid arthritis is symmetric, that is, there is circumferential narrowing of the joint. When large joints are affected (that is, knee), it manifests as a uniformly narrowed joint space.

TEST RATIONALE
MRI can be a useful clinical tool for showing the extent of disease. In the past it was felt unnecessary to perform MRI in the setting of rheumatoid arthritis. Pannus cannot be reliably differentiated from synovium and joint fluid; however, with gadolinium some investigators have reported that pannus (soft tissue thickening) can be easily identified because of the intense enhancement that occurs. Rheumatologists have become more aggressive and MRI is often performed for evaluation of pannus to help determine a treatment plan, as well as response to treatment (see Figs. 7-3A and 7-3B).

TEST OF CHOICE
Initial diagnosis: conventional radiography.
Response to treatment: MRI.

BIBLIOGRAPHY
Kaplan P, Helms CA, Dussault R, Anderson MW, Major NM. *Musculoskeletal MRI*. Philadelphia, PA: W.B. Saunders, 2001.
Smith HR. "Rheumatoid Arthritis." eMedicine. June 19, 2008. Available at http://www.emedicine.com/med/topic2024.htm

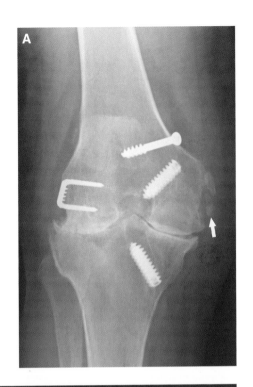

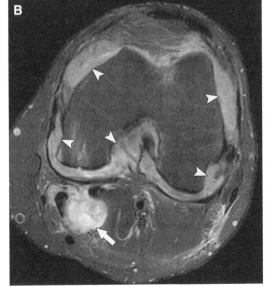

Figure 7-3   Rheumatoid arthritis. (A) Anterioposterior view of the knee demonstrates screw fixation consistent with anterior cruciate ligament (ACL) repair, medial collateral ligament injury (arrow) and lateral collateral ligament repair. Note the medial and lateral joint spaces are uniformly narrowed. Uniform, symmetric, joint-space narrowing is a finding that is seen with rheumatoid arthritis. (B) Axial T2 image demonstrating pannus (arrowheads) throughout the joint space.

7-4. Soft Tissue Tumor

CASE HISTORY

A 42-year-old female presents with history of soft tissue swelling in the hand unrelated to trauma.

BACKGROUND

Soft tissue tumors are a large and diverse group of neoplasms. Benign soft tissue tumors are common and usually treated with surgery alone when surgical resection is indicated. Before the 1970s, surgical resection was the primary therapy for malignant soft tissue tumors, and most patients with high-grade tumors had a poor prognosis and a considerable mortality rate. Since the mid-1970s, radiation therapy, chemotherapy, and advanced surgical techniques have helped increase long-term survival and decrease the need for ablative surgery. The most common symptom of a soft tissue tumor is a mass. It is usually painless and does not cause limb dysfunction. However, depending on the anatomic location of the tumor, it may cause pain or neurologic symptoms by irritating overlying bursae, compressing or stretching nerves, or by expanding sensitive structures. A rapid rate of increase in the size of a mass should arouse suspicion that the lesion is malignant or that hemorrhage has occurred in the lesion.

TEST RATIONALE

In the past 20 years, imaging studies have greatly contributed to the management of soft tissue tumors. MRI plays a central role in the work-up of a patient presenting with a suspected musculoskeletal tumor. MRI can confirm the presence of a lesion; allow for a specific diagnosis (in some cases); define the extent of tumor spread; provide biopsy guidance; and assist in the evaluation of recurrent disease after therapy (see Figs. 7-4A and 7-4B). In the patient with a suspected soft tissue mass, conventional radiographs still should be obtained because they may reveal bone involvement or soft tissue calcifications that might be helpful in the evaluation and not seen on MRI. In some cases, the MR appearance of a soft tissue mass is so characteristic that a confident, specific diagnosis can be provided, obviating further work-up. Even if the MR features do not allow a specific diagnosis to be made, MRI is still useful for evaluation of the extent of the lesion. In the setting of superimposed hemorrhage, the mass should be followed clinically or with MR to resolution.

TEST OF CHOICE

Conventional radiograph followed by MRI.

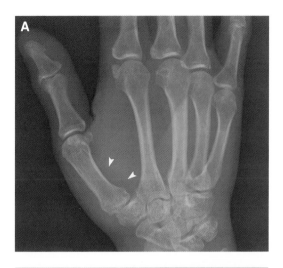

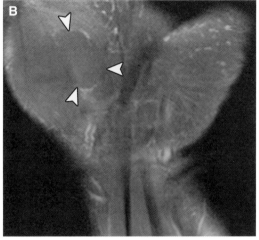

Figure 7-4 Soft tissue tumor. Palpable mass in the hand. (A) Anterioposterior view of the hand demonstrates fat density adjacent to the first metacarpal (arrowheads). (B) Coronal fat suppressed image through the hand demonstrates homogeneous suppression of the mass. The imaging characteristics are classic for a lipoma (fatty mass).

BIBLIOGRAPHY

Kaplan P, Helms CA, Dussault R, Anderson MW, Major NM. *Musculoskeletal MRI.* 1st edition, Philadelphia, PA: W. B. Saunders, 2001.

Shidham VB. "Benign and Malignant Soft Tissue Tumors." eMedicine. April 10, 2008 Available at http://www.emedicine.com/orthoped/TOPIC377.HTM

7-5. Rotator Cuff Tear

CASE HISTORY
A 46-year-old patient presents with history of prior shoulder dislocation and persistent pain.

BACKGROUND
The glenohumeral joint is the most mobile in the body. Its stability is due, in large part, to two structures: the rotator cuff and the glenoid labrum. The muscles of the rotator cuff pull the head of the humerus into the glenoid fossa while the fibrocartilaginous labrum serves to deepen the shallow glenoid fossa, increasing its surface area. The rotator cuff is comprised of four large tendons and is formed by the confluence of four muscles that originate on the scapula and insert on the humeral head: the supraspinatous, infraspinatous, teres minor, and subscapularis. Etiologies of rotator cuff tears (tear in one of the tendons) can be due to acute events or chronic degeneration. Impingement syndromes (the acrominon rubbing on the cuff) are a major cause of rotator cuff pathology in patients aged over 40 years. In addition to the rotator cuff, injuries to the glenoid labrum are also a common cause of shoulder pain, pathology, and instability and likewise can be due to chronic degeneration or acute injury. Injuries to the glenoid labrum disrupt the continuity of this fibrocartilaginous ring at various sites along its circumference leading to pain and instability.

TEST RATIONALE
In the acute setting of trauma, MRI with contrast is not necessary because there is generally enough fluid in the joint space to make a diagnosis of a labral tear or ligamentous injury (see Fig. 7-5A). For chronic injuries injection of intra-articular contrast, which fills the joint spaces with bright signal fluid, is helpful in delineating subtle injuries, especially posterior labral tears and labral-ligamentous tears (see Fig. 7-5B). Mimics of rotator cuff pathology, such as nerve entrapment syndromes, can also be diagnosed on MR images. Ultrasound is an alternative examination for the shoulder and rotator cuff. An accurate examination requires an expert sonographer. Because of the small field of view, often only a single structure can be evaluated in one ultrasound image. For example, labral detail cannot be assessed at the time the rotator cuff is being evaluated.

TEST OF CHOICE
In the acute setting: noncontrast MRI.
In the patient with chronic pain: MRI with intra-articular contrast.

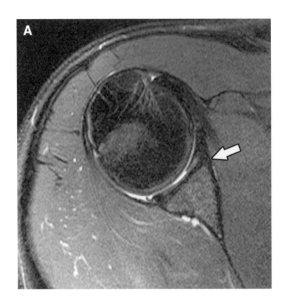

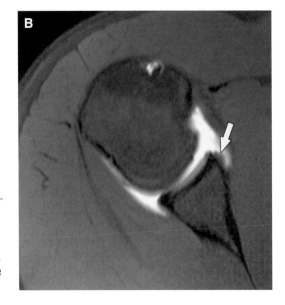

Figure 7-5 History of anterior shoulder dislocation. (A) Noncontrast (conventional MRI) axial T2 image shows normal low signal triangular shaped anterior (arrow) and posterior labrum. (B) Axial fat suppressed image with dilute gadolinium solution in the joint space shows displaced labrum (arrow) not seen on the noncontrast study. MRI, magnetic resonance imaging.

BIBLIOGRAPHY

American Academy of Orthopaedic Surgeons. "Rotator Cuff Tears: Frequently Asked Questions". April 10, 2008. Available at http://ortho-info.aaos.org/topic.cfm?topic=A00378

Tuite M. Shoulder, Rotator Cuff Injury (MRI). eMedicine. June 19, 2008. Available at http://www.emedicine.com/radio/topic894.htm

7-6. Cervical Spine Injury

CASE HISTORY
A 35-year-old male in a motor vehicle accident, ejected from car with suspected neck injury is brought in by ambulance to the emergency room.

BACKGROUND
Approximately 1 million people per year are admitted to U.S. emergency departments for injuries to the cervical spine. The incidence of acute fracture or major spinal injury, however, is less than 1%. Yet, missing an injury that compromises the spinal cord could be catastrophic.

TEST RATIONALE
In the past, patients with trauma to the cervical spine have traditionally been evaluated with conventional radiographs. The shortcoming of this approach is the difficulty in adequately visualizing the proximal and distal cervical regions. It has been shown that conventional radiographs can miss up to 50% of spine fractures that were ultimately discovered by computed tomography (CT). The advantage of CT is that it allows faster exclusion of injuries, expedites patient management, and detects more injuries than conventional radiography. CT, however, is only the test of choice in moderate-to high-risk patients. High-risk patients have sustained severe head trauma, have focal neurologic deficits, and/or a high-energy mechanism of injury (that is, car accident) (see Figs. 7-6A and 7-6B). Low-risk patients, those who are conscious, can undergo physical examination and have undergone a low- to moderate-energy trauma should first undergo examination with conventional radiography. The lateral film in particular is useful in assessing soft tissue swelling and vertebral alignment.

TEST OF CHOICE
Because this patient sustained a high-energy mechanism of injury, CT is the test of choice. In fact, in this high-risk trauma patient, CT would be the test of choice to evaluate injuries to the head, chest, abdomen, and pelvis.

BIBLIOGRAPHY
Blackmore CC, Emerson SS, Mann FA, Koepsell TD. Cervical spine imaging in patients with trauma: determination of fracture risk to optimize use. *Radiology*. 1999;211:759-765.
Stiell IG, Wells GA, Vandemheen KL, et al. The Canadian C-spine rule for radiography in alert and stable trauma patients. *JAMA*. 2001;286: 1841-1848.

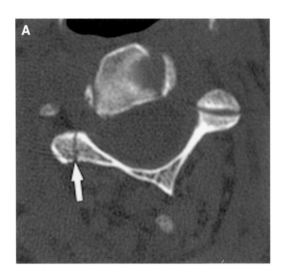

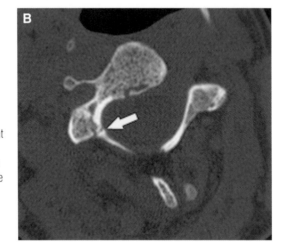

Figure 7-6   C-spine injury. History of motor vehicle crash and neck pain. Lateral C-spine demonstrating visualization of seven cervical vertebrae except for inferior aspect of C-7. Slight straightening of alignment (a nonspecific finding) and no significant soft tissue swelling. Two consecutive axial images through the cervical spine demonstrating a nondisplaced fracture through the facet (A) and lamina (B) (arrows).

7-7. Knee Injury

CASE HISTORY
A 25-year-old male presents with joint swelling and vague knee pain.

BACKGROUND
Knee injuries are the most common complaint seen by orthopedic surgeons. Cartilage pathology is one the most common findings in this subset of patients. There are two different types of cartilage present in the knee: the menisci (fibrocartilage) and articular cartilage (hyaline). The menisci (lateral and medial) are two C-shaped, cartilaginous structures found between the femur and tibial plateau that function to increase surface area and reduce friction during movement. Articular cartilage is found on the end of bones at the joint. These two structures are important for many of the functions of the knee joint including cushioning, friction free gliding of the femur on the tibia, weight distribution, and multidirectional movement. The etiology of cartilage injures can be attributed to both acute trauma and chronic degeneration. Symptoms associated with injury to the meniscus include joint line tenderness, swelling and stiffness, catching and locking of the knee, and knee buckling ("giving out").

TEST RATIONALE
Perhaps the biggest change in the past few years in musculoskeletal imaging has been in the area of cartilage evaluation. Every knee magnetic resonance (MR) examination should have a cartilage-sensitive sequence. Articular cartilage treatment has become important in orthopedic surgery and MRI is known to be useful in demonstrating abnormal cartilage in the knee, ankle, and elbow. Articular cartilage thickness seems to be dependent on patient age and activity level. When evaluating MR images all hyaline cartilage surfaces need to be inspected for pathology. We have found that it is preferable to have a cartilage-sensitive sequence in all three planes (axial, sagittal, coronal) because the abnormality may be more readily identified in one of the planes and subtle (or unseen) in the other two (see Figs. 7-7A and 7-7B). It should be noted that the patellar cartilage is generally thicker than the cartilage found on the femoral condyle and the tibial plateau.

TEST OF CHOICE
Noncontrast MRI.

BIBLIOGRAPHY
American Academy of Orthopaedic Surgeons. "Meniscal Tear". April 10, 2008. Available at http://orthoinfo.aaos.org/topic.cfm?topic=A00358
Kaplan P, Helms CA, Dussault R, Anderson MW, Major NM. *Musculoskeletal MRI*. Philadelphia, PA: W. B. Saunders, 2001.

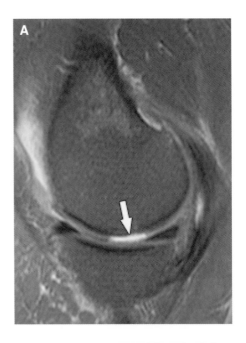

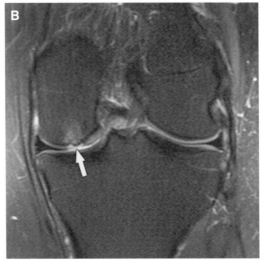

Figure 7-7   Cartilage injury. Sagittal (A) and coronal (B) images demonstrate a focal full thickness hyaline cartilage abnormality (arrows). Cartilage is intermediate in signal. The defect is filled with joint fluid (high signal).

7-8. Knee Dislocation

CASE HISTORY
A 30-year-old male in head-on collision motor vehicle accident, with swollen and stiff knee presents to the emergency department.

BACKGROUND
Knee dislocation is a rare event but important to recognize because it is often associated with a vascular injury to the popliteal artery and if not detected can lead to loss of the affected limb. The diagnosis is complicated by the fact that knee dislocation often presents in the context of spontaneous relocation or multisystem trauma so it can be over looked. Because the knee is a very stable joint and at least three major ligaments must rupture for the knee to dislocate, and it is therefore most often seen in high-energy trauma. Clinically, the affected limb usually has a gross deformity about the knee with swelling and immobility. Because of the high incidence of vascular and neurologic injury, evaluation of these structures is essential.

TEST RATIONALE
There are two major concerns in this scenario: evaluation of the ligaments of the knee and assessment of the popliteal artery (see Figs. 7-8A and 7-8B). In the past, patients received both conventional angiography and MRI. The time required to move the patient from one radiology examination room to another and perform the tests was significant and could delay diagnosis. MRI can now be performed utilizing special sequences to evaluate arterial flow and ligaments during the same examination. Intravenous contrast material can be reserved for use in revascularization procedures.

TEST OF CHOICE
MR angiography.

BIBLIOGRAPHY
Green JR. "Knee Dislocation." eMedicine. June 19, 2008. Available at http://www.emedicine.com/orthoped/topic409.htm
Rihn JA, Groff YJ, Harner CD, Cha PS. The acutely dislocated knee: evaluation and management. *J Am Acad Orthop Surg*. 2004;12:335-336.

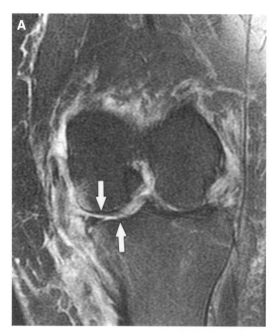

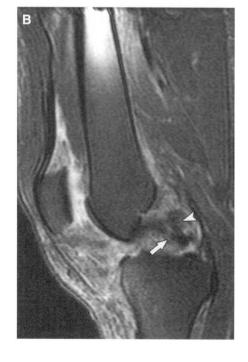

Figure 7-8 Knee dislocation. (A) Coronal image through the region of the notch demonstrates medial subluxation of the femur relative to the tibia (arrows). The MCL is torn. (B) Sagittal image through the notch demonstrates a torn ACL (not visualized) and a torn PCL (thickened and abnormal configuration). The arrow and arrowheads identify the abnormal ligaments within the notch. The bright area in the distal femur represents artifact from an intramedullary rod that was placed for a femur fracture.
ACL, anterior cruciate ligament; MCL, medial collateral ligament; PCL, posterior cruciate ligament.

7-9. Back Pain

CASE HISTORY
A 35-year-old construction worker presents with new-onset low back pain.

BACKGROUND
Back pain is extremely common. Almost all people will experience one episode of back pain in their lifetime. Low back pain is the leading cause of job-related disability and the second leading neurological ailment behind headaches in the United States. Back pain can range from acute to chronic (lasting >3 months). For patients younger than 45 years old, low back pain is usually secondary to a mechanical problem such as fracture, muscle spasm, or acute disc extrusion. Degenerative disease is the most common etiology of low back pain in patients greater than 45 years old. It must be noted that most symptoms of back pain are not related to nerve involvement but to the spine, muscles, or other structures in the back. Symptoms may range from limited flexibility and/or range of motion, muscle ache to shooting or stabbing pain, or an inability to stand straight. Most episodes of back pain can be conservatively managed and will resolve within 2–4 weeks.

TEST RATIONALE
Before imaging studies, the best diagnostic tool is a thorough history and physical examination, which are vital in evaluation, treatment, and management of lower back pain. There is a weak association between symptoms and imaging results. Imaging studies should only be ordered in patients with trauma or clinical findings suggestive of systemic disease (that is, patients older than 50 years, weight loss without explanation, fever, intravenous drug abuse, or alcohol use). The Quebec Task Force of Spinal Disorders suggests that early (<4 weeks) conventional radiographs are necessary only if the patient is older than 50 years or younger than 20 years, and has fever, neurologic deficits, trauma, or signs of neoplasm. Persistent mechanical lower back pain (>4 weeks) may require additional imaging studies including MRI, CT and/or 3-phase bone scan (see Figs. 7-9A, 7-9B, and 7-9C). MRI is superior to CT because of the greater soft tissue detail. Bone scan can be helpful in localizing metastatic disease of infection.

TEST OF CHOICE
Conventional radiography, then, MRI if refractory to supportive management.

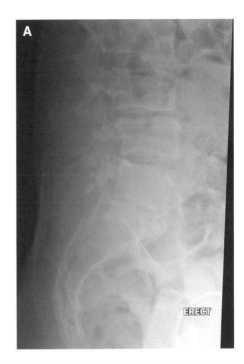

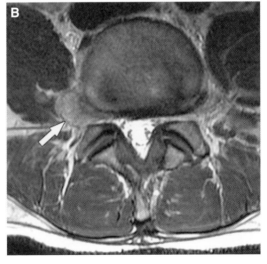

Figures 7-9 Disc disease versus muscle strain. (A) Lateral plain film shows disc space narrowing. The disc is not identified on a conventional x-ray (unless it is calcified). (B) Axial image through the L4–5 disc space level shows a far lateral protrusion of the disc in the foramen (arrow). MR is very helpful to identify where the disc is protruded and to explain the clinical findings of right L4 radiculopathy (affecting L4 in the foramen). (C) Far right sagittal image shows the disc protrusion in the foramen (arrow). MR, magnetic resonance.

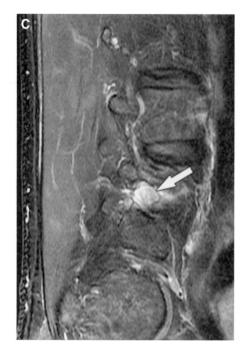

Figures 7-9   Continued.

BIBLIOGRAPHY
Atlas SJ, Deyo RA, Patrick DL, Convery K, Keller RB, Singer DE. The Quebec Task Force classification for Spinal Disorders and the severity, treatment, and outcomes of sciatica and lumbar spinal stenosis. *Spine.* 1996 Dec 15;21(24):2885-2892.
Hills EC. "Mechanical Low Back Pain." eMedicine. April 10, 2008. Available at http://www.emedicine.com/pmr/topic73.htm

7-10. Bone Tumors

CASE HISTORY
A 10-year-old male presents with onset of shoulder pain noted after mild trauma.

BACKGROUND
Primary malignant bone tumors are very rare, representing less than 1% of all malignant tumors and usually occur in young men between the ages of 10 and 20. However, not all primary bone tumors are malignant and some of these benign primary bone tumors will spontaneously resolve. Osteochondroma is the most common benign primary bone tumor. Malignant bone tumors include osteosarcomas, Ewing's sarcoma, fibrosarcoma, and chondrosarcoma. Ewing's sarcoma can arise anywhere in the body, but has a predilection for the long bones of the legs and arms, the chest, or the pelvis. Usually the symptoms are few, the most common being pain and swelling at the site of the tumor Children may also present with pathologic fractures or have a history of fever. Approximately 30% of children will have metastatic disease (to lung and bone) at the time of diagnosis.

TEST RATIONALE
Conventional radiography is necessary to characterize a lesion in the bone as benign or aggressive based primarily upon its margins. Additional characteristics that are evaluated include internal characteristics of the lesion and associated densities (see Fig. 7-10A). MRI may reveal margins that are difficult to characterize (see Fig. 7-10B). Edema, as well as soft tissue components, can be seen with benign or aggressive processes. So the characterization on plain film is imperative before the MR is performed. For malignant processes the MR is useful for staging and assessing adjacent neurovascular structures.

MR is not useful in the initial diagnosis of Ewing's sarcoma. The characteristic findings of the wide zone of transition, permeative process, and aggressive periosteal reaction are seen on conventional radiography with all primary sarcomas of bone. MR can help identify missed lesions and is useful in staging.

TEST OF CHOICE
Conventional radiography.

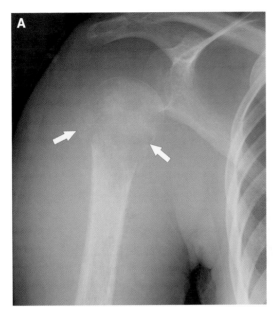

Figures 7-10   Primary bone tumor, Ewing's sarcoma. (A) Anterioposterior radiograph of the proximal humerus shows a permeative process, wide zone of transition (aggressive features) with pathologic fracture (arrows) in the proximal metaphysis of the humerus. (B) Coronal MRI image through the humerus shows significant soft tissue mass along with abnormal signal within the bone. The MRI appearance is not specific for a Ewing's sarcoma.
MRI, magnetic resonance imaging.

BIBLIOGRAPHY
Nanda R. "Bone Tumors." Medline Plus. April 10, 2008. Available at http://www.nlm.nih.gov/medlineplus/ency/article/001230.htm
Strauss LG. "Ewing Sarcoma." eMedicine. June 19, 2008. Available at http://www.emedicine.com/radio/topic275.htm

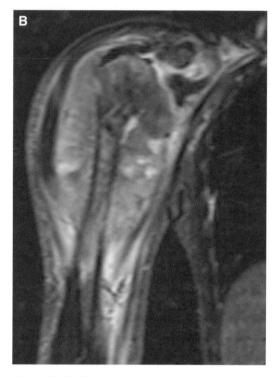

Figures 7-10   Continued.

8

DISEASES OF THE CARDIOVASCULAR SYSTEM

W. Brian Hyslop and Robert Dixon

8-1. Back Pain

CASE HISTORY
A 56-year-old male presents with hypertension and sudden onset searing back pain.

BACKGROUND
Aortic dissection originates as a tear in the aortic intima. It most commonly originates in the ascending aorta or the region of the ligamentum arteriosum. Propagation of the dissection results in the formation of a false lumen. Type A dissection involves the ascending aorta while Type B aortic dissection involves the aorta distal to the origin of the left subclavian artery. Abrupt onset of knife-like chest pain is the most common presenting symptom. Aortic dissection has an incidence of 5–30 cases per million people per year with 80%–90% of patients greater than 60 years of age. Risk factors include hypertension, atherosclerosis, and underlying aortic diseases.

TEST RATIONALE
Contrast-enhanced computed tomography (CT) or magnetic resonance angiography (MRA) is the study of choice to evaluate the presence and extent of aortic dissection (see Figs. 8-1A and 8-1B). Their multiplanar imaging capabilities are well suited to assessing the proximal extent of the dissection, which is critical in planning surgical versus medical management. In addition, both may detect complications of aortic dissection that include aortic rupture, hypoperfusion of vascular territories, and involvement of the aortic root (valve or coronary arteries). In the acute setting, CT angiography (CTA) may be performed more rapidly. In younger patients with predisposing conditions, such as Turner or Marfan syndrome, MRA may be preferred due to the lack of ionizing radiation.

TEST OF CHOICE
CTA or MRA.

BIBLIOGRAPHY
Chaughtai A, Kazerooni EA. CT and MRI of acute thoracic cardiovascular emergencies. *Crit Care Clin.* 2007;23:835-853.
Shiga T, Wajima Z, Apfel CC, Inoue T, Ohe Y. Diagnostic accuracy of transesophageal echocardiography, helical computed tomography, and magnetic resonance imaging for suspected thoracic aortic dissection: systematic review and meta-analysis. *Arch Intern Med.* 2006 Jul 10;166(13):1350-1356.

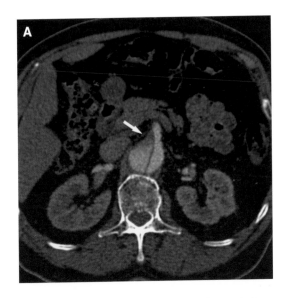

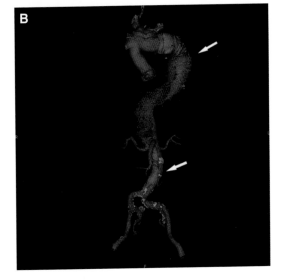

Figure 8-1 (A) Axial-contrast CT shows the dissection flap (black line) extending into the superior mesenteric artery (arrow). (B) Reformatted image shows the dissection in blue extending from the subclavian artery to just above the aortic bifurcation (arrows). CT, computed tomography.

8-2. Screening for Coronary Artery Disease

CASE HISTORY
Asymptomatic obese male with hypertension.

BACKGROUND
Coronary artery disease is a leading cause of death in the industrialized world. The most common etiology is atherosclerotic disease with plaque formation. Plaque formation may result in luminal narrowing of a vessel, while plaque rupture with subsequent thrombosis may result in acute narrowing or occlusion of a coronary artery. Because approximately 50% of patients with coronary artery disease initially present with either an acute myocardial infarction or sudden cardiac death, methods for identifying people at increased risk for coronary artery disease are needed to identify people who may benefit from secondary prevention strategies.

TEST RATIONALE
Identification of patients at risk for coronary artery disease may begin with a Framingham risk score evaluation. For those patients at intermediate risk based on this evaluation, further risk stratification may be done using techniques such as electrocardiographic stress testing or calcium scoring. Calcium scoring is a noncontrast electrocardiographically gated CT of the heart that can quantitatively measure the amount of atherosclerotic calcification within the coronary arteries (see Figs. 8-2A and 8-2B). With the establishment of normal ranges of coronary calcium as a function of age, gender, and ethnicity, calcium scoring has been shown to result in improved identification of patients at risk for a sudden cardiac event. Thus, calcium scoring may aid in identifying subjects with underlying coronary artery disease that would benefit from more aggressive pharmacologic or lifestyle intervention.

TEST OF CHOICE
Calcium scoring.

BIBLIOGRAPHY
Detrano R, Guerci AD, Carr JJ, et al. Coronary Calcium as a Predictor of Coronary Events in Four Racial or Ethnic Groups. *N Engl J Med.* 2008;358:1336-1345.

Greenland P, Labree L, Azen SP, Doherty TM, Detrano RC. Coronary artery calcium score combined with Framingham score for risk prediction in asymptomatic individuals. *JAMA.* 2004;291:210-215.

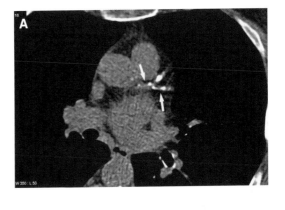

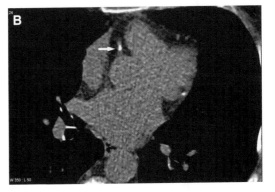

Figure 8-2
(A) Noncontrast axial image of the heart demonstrates multiple sites of atherosclerotic calcification in the left coronary arterial circulation. (B) Noncontrast axial image of the heart more inferiorly demonstrates atherosclerotic calcification in the right coronary artery.

8-3. Persistent Heart failure following Myocardial Infarction

CASE HISTORY
A 73-year-old male with myocardial infarction 3 months ago who now presents with persistent symptoms of heart failure.

BACKGROUND
Long-term consequences of myocardial infarction include abnormalities in left ventricular contractility, development of arrhythmias, and mitral valvular dysfunction secondary to the infarct itself or ventricular remodeling. The mortality from congestive heart failure has more than doubled during the time period 1970–2000. Differentiation of myocardial ischemia from either full-thickness (transmural) or partial-thickness (subendocardial or nontransmural) myocardial infarct may aid in the determination of surgical versus nonsurgical management. If surgery is indicated, information on the extent of infarct will also aid in selection of the type of surgery.

TEST RATIONALE
Nuclear stress imaging, stress echocardiography, and cardiac MRI have all been utilized for the assessment of cardiac viability (see Figs. 8-3A and 8-3B). Cardiac MRI has the advantage of assessing for viability, valvular disease, and cardiac function during one examination. Following the administration of gadolinium-based MRI contrast, contrast over time (>15 minutes) will preferentially sequester within the infarct resulting in bright signal. The normally perfused heart will remain dark. The sensitivity of contrast-enhanced cardiac MRI to subendocardial infarction is superior to that of thallium-based scans, and correlates closely with results of positron emission tomography (PET). Increased sensitivity is of particular value in diabetic patients who may suffer from occult infarcts. It has been shown that the utility of a revascularization procedure, such as coronary artery bypass graft surgery, decreases with increasing wall thickness of the infarct as determined by MRI.

TEST OF CHOICE
Contrast-enhanced MRI.

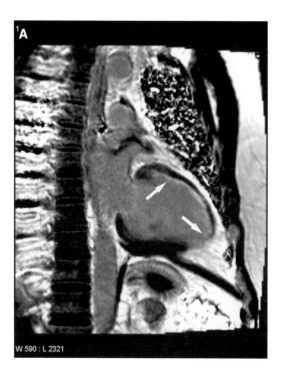

Figure 8-3 (A) Postcontrast delayed hyperenhancement two-chamber view of the left ventricle demonstrating a subendocardial and transmural regions of hyperenhancement in the anterior wall. (B) Short-axis image in the apex demonstrates a transmural infarct in the apical region of the left ventricle with nonenhancing apical thrombus (arrow).

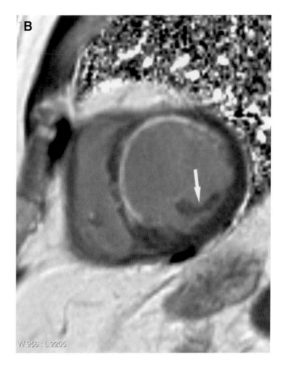

Figure 8-3   Continued.

BIBLIOGRAPHY

Kim RJ, Wu E, Rafael A, et al. The use of contrast-enhanced magnetic resonance imaging to identify reversible myocardial dysfunction. *N Engl J Med.* 2000;343:1445-1453.

Thomson LE, Kim RJ, Judd RM. Magnetic resonance imaging for the assessment of myocardial viability. *JMRI.* 2004;19:771-788.

8-4. Episodic Chest Pain

CASE HISTORY
A 50-year-old woman presents with occasional episodes of chest pain.

BACKGROUND
Chest pain is the most common presenting symptom in patients with obstructive coronary artery disease. The differential for chest pain includes cardiac, pulmonary, gastrointestinal, and musculoskeletal etiologies.

TEST RATIONALE
Depending on its acuity, the initial work-up may include electrocardiography (ECG), chest radiography, and image-based stress testing. Although a noncontrast calcium scoring study may identify subjects at increased risk for coronary artery disease, it is insensitive to both noncalcified atherosclerotic plaque and flow-limiting lesions in the symptomatic patient. However, the high negative predictive value of contrast-enhanced cardiac CTA makes it useful in the low- to intermediate-risk patient to exclude obstructive coronary artery disease (see Figs. 8-4A and 8-4B), particularly in those patients with uninterpretable ECG or who are unable to exercise. It may be used in patients with nondiagnostic stress imaging tests to exclude obstructive coronary artery disease. Finally, several studies have suggested that in the acute setting, coronary CTA may be used in lieu of stress testing in the low- to intermediate-risk patient to more rapidly exclude coronary artery disease.

TEST OF CHOICE
CTA in patients with an intermediate test probability who are either unable to exercise or have an uninterpretable ECG.

BIBLIOGRAPHY
Budoff MJ, Achenbach S, Blumenthal RS, et al. Assessment of coronary artery disease by cardiac computed tomography: a scientific statement. *Circulation*. 2006;114:1761-1791.

Schoenhagen P, Halliburton SS, Stillman AE, et al. Noninvasive imaging of coronary arteries: current and future role of multi-detector row CT. *Radiology*. 2004;232:7-17.

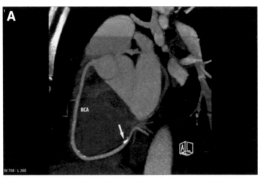

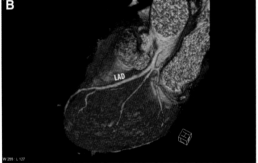

Figure 8-4
(A) Maximum intensity projection (MIP) of the right coronary artery (RCA) demonstrates atherosclerotic calcium in its distal aspect. (B) MIP of the proximal left coronary arterial system demonstrates eccentric calcification in the proximal left anterior descending coronary artery (LAD) and less than 50% stenosis in an intermediate ramus.

8-5. Sudden Cardiac Death

CASE HISTORY
A healthy 12-year-old male collapses during a basketball game.

BACKGROUND
Within the United States, there are roughly 500 deaths per year in the pediatric population secondary to sudden cardiac death. Although the etiology of cardiogenic syncope in the pediatric patient is more commonly neurally mediated, features of the event history (syncope during exertion, without prodrome, or with associated cardiac event) as well as family history warrant further work-up. Cardiac etiologies with a morphologic correlate include cardiomyopathies, congenital cardiac anomalies (including anomalous coronary arteries), and arrhythmogenic right ventricular dysplasia (ARVD).

TEST RATIONALE
Echocardiography is commonly the first imaging study used to assess for structural abnormalities. A cardiac catheterization may be performed to exclude anomalous coronary artery anomalies. However, a contrast-enhanced cardiac MRI can assess both morphology and function of the heart, the presence of anomalous origins of the coronary arteries (although evaluation for luminal narrowing in the coronary arterial tree is more commonly performed with contrast-enhanced cardiac CT), and is the imaging modality of choice for the assessment of wall dysplasia (see Figs. 8-5A and 8-5B).

TEST OF CHOICE
Cardiac MRI.

BIBLIOGRAPHY
Sudden Cardiac Death in Children and Adolescents. Guest Editor—Stuart Berger. Pediatric Clinics of North America. 2004;51:1201-1463.
Johnsrude CL. Current approach to pediatric syncope. *Pediatr Cardiol.* 2000;21:522-531.

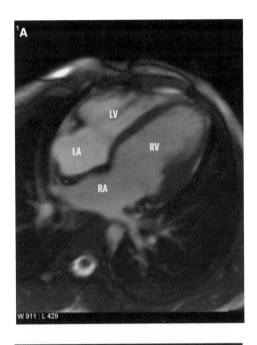

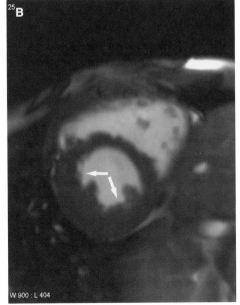

Figures 8-5 Short axis (A) and four-chamber (B) bright blood image of a 9-year-old patient resuscitated by AED following collapse during a recreational sports event demonstrates asymmetric wall thickening in the basilar lateral wall during diastole. No abnormal enhancement was noted to suggest infiltrative disease. The findings were suggestive of hypertrophic cardiomyopathy.
AED, automated external defibrillator.

8-6. Severe Hypertension

CASE HISTORY
A 68-year-old male presents with new onset of severe hypertension and flash pulmonary edema.

BACKGROUND
The vast majority of hypertensive patients have primary or essential hypertension. However, secondary hypertension due to renal artery stenosis (RAS) accounts for a small (<5%), but important group of all hypertensive patients. The importance of diagnosing RAS is that it is a potentially treatable cause (of both hypertension and renal insufficiency) that responds to interventions, such as renal artery angioplasty, stenting, or open surgery. However, only those patients with a clinical scenario compatible with a vascular etiology should undergo screening. These include patients with a sudden onset of severe hypertension or sudden worsening of hypertension, onset of hypertension in a young patient (<30 years) or an older adult (>50 years), and hypertension poorly controlled by three antihypertensive agents.

TEST RATIONALE
The imaging of RAS is a complex issue involving multiple clinical factors and various patient populations. There is no one test that is ideal for all patients, as age, renal function, prior surgical history, and suspected etiology all play a role in imaging selection. The most common etiology of RAS is atherosclerotic disease involving the origin of the main renal artery. Ultrasound lacks reproducibility and is rarely used. Renal scintigraphy has been shown to be sensitive and specific in adults with normal renal function and unilateral disease; however, many patients do not fit these criteria and this study does not provide anatomic detail. MRA and CTA are widely available and accurate, with sensitivities and specificities on the order of 100% and 94% (see Fig. 8-6A). CTA requires the use of iodinated-contrast agent and uses ionizing radiation. When compared to MRA, CTA has the advantages of improved-spatial resolution, decreased total examination time, and better ability to evaluate the patency of indwelling stents. The absence of radiation in MRA is an appealing characteristic. Historically, MR was thought to be safe in patients with renal insufficiency or failure; however, nephrogenic systemic fibrosis (NSF), a systemic disorder that predominately affects the skin, has been linked with gadolinium-based contrast agents and patients with renal failure. Digital subtracted angiography (DSA) should be reserved for cases where intervention is planned or where

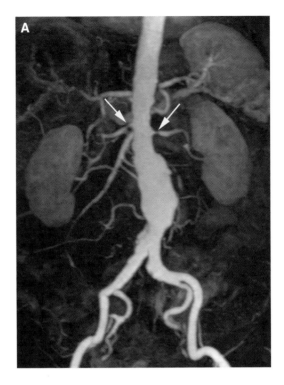

Figure 8-6   (A) MIP image from 3D–contrast-enhanced MRA reveals bilateral renal artery stenoses (arrows) and an infra-renal abdominal aortic aneurysm. (B1) DSA aorto-gram demonstrates a diffusely narrowed aorta with stenoses of two right renal arteries and a single left renal artery (arrowheads) in a 3-year-old female with malignant hypertension who presented with intracranial hemorrhage. A prominent inferior mesenteric artery feed-ing the Arc of Riolan (collateral supply to the stenotic superior mesenteric artery) is seen as well (arrow). (B2) She eventually went on to have surgery with re-implantation of her renal arteries , which significantly improved her hypertension, allowing her to recover completely from her intracranial hemorrhage. Pathology identified this as fibromuscular dysplasia. DSA, digital subtraction arteriography; MIP, maximum intensity projection; MRA, magnetic resonance angiography.

confirmation is required (see Figs. 8-6B1 and 8-6B2). A special note should be made of younger patients. Pediatric patients with hypertension will require DSA for evaluation, as they may have subtle stenoses involving the distal branches of the renal artery or an accessory renal artery.

TEST OF CHOICE
- MRA.
- CTA if not MR compatible, evaluation of renal artery stent or concern for NSF.
- DSA if pediatric patient or for confirmation/planned intervention.

BIBLIOGRAPHY
Glockner JF, Vrtiska TJ. Renal MR and CT angiography: current concepts. *Abdom Imaging*. 2007;32:407-420.

Vo NJ, Hammelman BD, Racadio JM, Stife CF, Johnson ND, Racadio JM. Anatomic distribution of renal artery stenosis in children: implications for imaging. *Pediatr Radiol*. 2006;36:1032-1036.

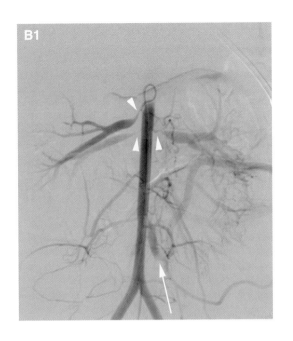

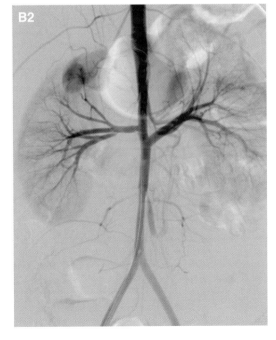

Figure 8-6 Continued.

8-7. Asymptomatic Patient following Abdominal Aortic Aneurysm Repair

CASE HISTORY

A 68-year-old male presents with increasing size of aneurysm following endovascular repair of abdominal aortic aneurysm.

BACKGROUND

Since it was first performed in 1991, endovascular aneurysm repair (EVAR) has become a viable alternative to open surgical repair in select cases. The advantage of an endovascular approach is the diminished morbidity and mortality associated with this procedure when compared to an open repair; the disadvantage is that life long imaging is required to search for various complications, including endoleaks (blood flow outside the lumen of the endograft, but within the lumen of the native aneurysm). Endoleaks occur in approximately one-quarter of endovascular repairs, but have been reported in as many as 44% of cases. However, endoleaks do not occur following open surgical repair. Endoleaks can be divided into five different types based on the source of the leak

Type I: involve the proximal (IA) or distal (IB) attachment sites.

Type II: secondary to flow from branch vessels, such as the inferior mesenteric artery or lumbar arteries. This is the most common type of endoleak and can be further divided into those involving only one vessel (IIA or "simple"), and those involving more than one vessel (IIB or "complex") (see Fig. 8-7A).

Type III: graft failure secondary disruption of the body of the graft or detachment of its components (see Fig. 8-7B).

Type IV: graft porosity.

Type V: endotension—the continued increase in size of the native aneurysm sac, without identification of an endoleak.

Types I and III are less common, but they result in a direct pressurization of the native aneurysm sac, are associated with a significant risk of rupture, and should be treated immediately upon diagnosis. Type II endoleaks are the most common type following EVAR of abdominal aortic aneurysms, but many resolve spontaneously. However, persistent type II endoleaks that are associated with aneurysm enlargement are usually treated. Type IV leaks are not commonly seen with current materials used in endografts.

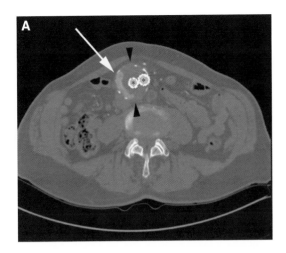

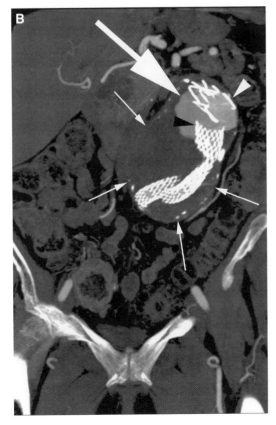

Figure 8-7 (A) Type II endoleak A type II endoleak is identified (white arrow) within the periphery of the native aneurysm sac (arrowheads). The two limbs of the endograft are seen (*) as well.
(B) Type III endoleak the proximal (white arrowhead) and distal (black arrowhead) components of the endograft have separated, resulting in a type III endoleak (large white arrow) which is seen within the native aneurysm sac (small white arrows).

TEST RATIONALE

Multiple imaging modalities (CTA, DSA, US, MRI, and plain films/radiographs) are involved in endoleak surveillance. CTA, typically using unenhanced, arterial, and delayed venous phase images, has become the imaging modality of choice at most institutions, primarily because of its widespread availability, noninvasive nature, rapid acquisition, ease of reproducibility and its lack of significant artifact from the endografts. The potential impact of the ionizing radiation involved in prolonged CTA surveillance has prompted some authors to recommend eliminating at least one of the three phases described earlier; thus, there is no consensus regarding the optimal CTA protocol. CTA has been shown to be more sensitive than angiography; however, once an endoleak is identified, angiography may be required to correctly classify the leak and possibly to repair it. Ultrasound is portable, noninvasive, safe, and inexpensive; it also does not involve ionizing radiation or potentially nephrotoxic contrast agents. MRA is also used and has been shown to be as sensitive (if not more sensitive) than CTA; however, certain endografts, which have a stainless steel framework, are considered to be non-MRI compatible and cause significant ferromagnetic artifact. Plain radiographs are also used in endoleak surveillance, as they assist with identifying subtle disruptions in the endograft framework (which may not be appreciated on CTA) and allow an overall view of the endograft's position and conformation.

TEST OF CHOICE
CTA.

BIBLIOGRAPHY

Kranokpiraksa P, Kaufman JA. Follow-up of endovascular aneurysm repair: plain radiography, ultrasound, CT/CT angiography, MR Imaging/MR angiography, or what? *J Vasc Interv Radiol.* 2008;19:S27-S36.

Stavropolos SW, Charagundla SR. Imaging Techniques for detection and management of endoleaks after endovascular aortic aneurysm repair. *Radiology.* 2007;243:641-655.

8-8. Claudication

CASE HISTORY
A 69-year-old diabetic presents with rest pain which has progressed to tissue loss.

BACKGROUND
Peripheral arterial disease (PAD) often presents initially with intermittent claudication, ischemic pain in the lower extremities, which is often described as a cramping, burning, or tightness that occurs with exertion and is relieved by rest. Risk factors for PAD include advanced age, smoking, diabetes, hypertension, and hyperlipidemia. As the severity of PAD progresses, the patient may experience ischemic rest pain, minor tissue loss (nonhealing ulcer) or major tissue loss. The initial evaluation of a patient with suspected PAD must include a detailed history and physical examination (as other pathologic processes can mimic claudication, most commonly neurogenic lower extremity pain) followed by noninvasive physiologic tests. If these indicate the presence of PAD, imaging may be initiated to plan anticipated revascularization. In addition, noninvasive therapies should be considered, including regular exercise, dietary modification, smoking cessation programs, antilipid agents, and antiplatelet agents.

TEST RATIONALE
After a detailed physical examination, noninvasive tests, including ankle-brachial index (ABI, the ration of the systolic ankle blood pressure to the arm blood pressure) and plethysmography, can be used to help confirm the presence of vascular disease and identify the general location of the disease process (inflow, outflow, or run-off disease). Once it has been determined that invasive therapy may be warranted, imaging will be required. While digital subtraction angiography (DSA) has long been considered the gold standard by which all other imaging modalities are measured, it is an invasive study with a small, but real risk of complications. Therefore, it is being displaced by increasingly robust noninvasive studies, which are used to identify the vascular regions involved, characterize the nature of stenosis and occlusions, and plan the revascularization procedure. Thus, DSA is now reserved for cases where intervention is planned or for cases where noninvasive studies require confirmation (see Fig. 8-8A). Duplex sonography, with a sensitivity and specificity of 88% and 95%, respectively, offers the benefit of using no radiation or iodinated contrast, but is patient and operator dependent. In addition, when compared to duplex sonography,

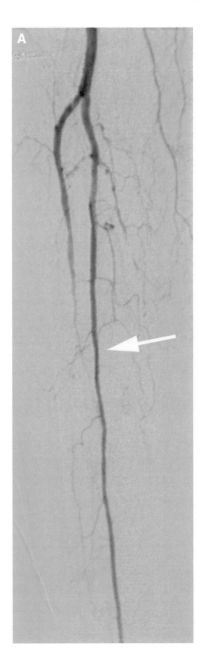

Figure 8-8 (A) Three-dimensional MIP image from an MRA of the right leg shows that the peroneal artery (arrow) is the only run-off vessel to the foot, while the anterior tibial artery (arrowhead) and posterior tibial artery (double arrowheads) occlude proximally. (B) DSA of the same patient performed 2 weeks after the MRA in Figure 8-8A (during an attempt to improve the vascular supply to the foot) confirms that the peroneal artery (arrow) is the only run-off vessel to the foot.
DSA, digital subtraction arteriography; MIP, maximum intensity projection; MRA, magnetic resonance angiography.

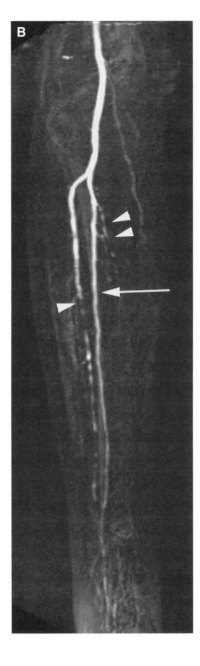

Figure 8-8 Continued.

recent studies have found both MRA and CTA to have slightly higher sensitivities (91%–98%) and specificities (92%–98%) and both to be more clinically useful, in that they result in higher diagnostic confidence and require less additional imaging (see Fig. 8-8B). CTA offers cost savings over MRA (1), but requires potentially nephrotoxic contrast and radiation to be used. In addition, heavily calcified arteries, particularly in the small run-off vessels below the knee, can be difficult to evaluate with CTA. On the other hand, MRA requires more time to perform and may be difficult for patients with claustrophobia or contraindicated because of non-MRI compatible devices. Moreover, indwelling vascular stents or surgical clips may result in significant artifacts on MRA. CTA and MRA have both continued to each evolve technically. Multidetector CTA is widely available with 16 to 64 detector CT found in most institutions. Advances in MRA, including parallel imaging and three-dimensional time-resolved imaging, have resulted in substantial improvement in the quality of studies being performed, and a reduction in the study time required. The risk of NSF must be recognized in patients with renal insufficiency or failure when considering MRA.

TEST OF CHOICE
MRA or CTA.

BIBLIOGRAPHY
Ersoy H, Rybicki FJ. MR angiography of the lower extremities. *AJR.* 2008;190:1675-1684.

Ouwendijk R, de Vries M, Stijnen T, et al. Multicenter randomized controlled trial of the costs and effects of noninvasive diagnostic imaging in patients with peripheral arterial disease: The DIPAS Trial. *AJR.* 2008;190:1349-1357.

8-9. Leg Swelling

CASE HISTORY
A 25-year-old woman complains of leg swelling following a 12 hour transatlantic airplane flight.

BACKGROUND
Venous thromboembolism (VTE) is a common problem, which affects approximately 5% of people in their lifetime, and can be manifested by deep venous thrombosis (DVT) and/or pulmonary embolism (PE), which is highly lethal. The history and physical in such cases is fairly nonspecific. As a result, an integrated approach is often used for the diagnosis of DVT, which employs estimating the pretest likelihood using an established prediction model, obtaining a D-dimer assay, and noninvasive imaging.

TEST RATIONALE
A detailed history and physical examination must be performed, and if DVT remains a consideration, a validated prediction model can be combined with a D-dimer assay. As the D-dimer assay is a very sensitive, but nonspecific test, a low pretest probability combined with a negative D-dimer essentially rules out a DVT. Other strategies have combined the pretest probability with ultrasound, establishing that a negative ultrasound combined with a low pretest probability safely excludes DVT. Ultrasound has been established as the imaging study of choice for DVT, with a sensitivity of at least 94% for proximal DVT (although lower in the calf) and a specificity of 94%. Findings on ultrasound indicative of DVT include the absence of compressibility, abnormal flow dynamics, and visualization of thrombus (see Figs. 8-9A1 and 8-9A2). If the diagnosis of DVT is felt to be likely, a negative ultrasound with a negative D-dimer excludes DVT, while a negative ultrasound with a *positive* D-dimer warrants serial ultrasonography. MRV is an evolving modality that has recently been shown to have similar sensitivity and specificity as ultrasound. It can be used to evaluate the central veins, which are not directly imaged with ultrasound. Venography is typically only used when prior studies are equivocal, or when intervention is planned (thrombolysis, mechanical thrombectomy, venoplasty, stenting, or IVC filter insertion) (see Fig. 8-9B). Established indications for IVC filters include failure of anticoagulation, contraindication to anticoagulation, or complication from anticoagulation.

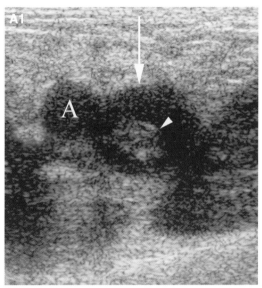

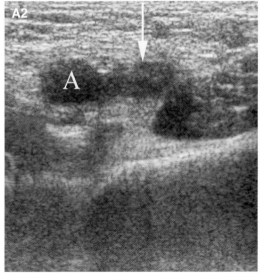

Figure 8-9 (A1) Ultrasound shows the common femoral vein (arrow) medial to the common femoral artery (A). Within the vein is an echogenic thrombus (arrowhead). (A2) With compression, the common femoral vein (arrow) is only partially compressible because of the thrombus. (B) Inferior venacavagram identifies a Günther Tulip IVC Filter (Cook Medical Inc., Bloomington, IN), which has been placed below the level of the renal veins, which are identified by the inflow of nonopacified blood (arrows). Note the hook on the filter (arrowhead) which allows the filter to be snared and retrieved.

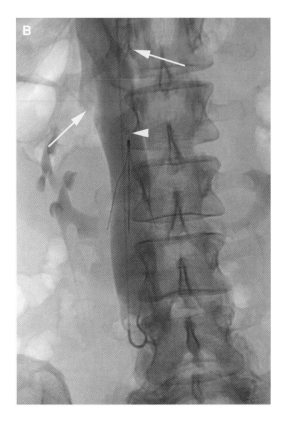

Figure 8-9   Continued.

TEST OF CHOICE
Ultrasound.

BIBLIOGRAPHY
Sampson FC, Goodacre SW, Thomas SM, van Beck EJR. The accuracy of
    MRI in diagnosis of suspected deep vein thrombosis: systemic review
    and meta-analysis. *Eur Radiol.* 2007;17:175-181.
Wells PS. Integrated strategies for the diagnosis of venous thromboembo-
    lism. *J Thromb Haemost.* 2007;5:41-50.

8-10. Dialysis Access

CASE HISTORY
A 58-year-old presents with a left arm fistula that has demonstrated decreased flow rates during dialysis.

BACKGROUND
Chronic kidney disease affects approximately 11% of adults in the United States, with an increasing incidence and prevalence of kidney failure, requiring over 300,000 people to receive some form of dialysis. Imaging is recommended for preoperative vascular mapping before placement of access (fistula or graft), and once access has been established, imaging and intervention will be required to maintain functioning access.

TEST RATIONALE
Ultrasound is the preferred method for preoperative vascular planning, as it can assess and map the peripheral arteries and veins. Patients with edema of an extremity, collateral vein development, differential extremity size, a pacemaker, current or previous catheter placement, or previous extremity, neck or chest trauma, should also undergo venography preoperatively to evaluate the central veins. MRV may also be used to evaluate central vessels. Once a fistula or graft is in place and is being used, various screening methods (physical examination, flow rates, pressures) will uncover access dysfunction (see Figs. 8-10A and 8-10B). This is most frequently evaluated by venography, as an intervention (angioplasty or stenting) is almost always required to treat the underlying lesion and maintain adequate dialysis access. If these measures are unsuccessful, surgical revision may be required. In the event of thrombosis of a graft or fistula, a percutaneous thrombectomy or thrombolysis can be performed to restore patency and also to treat the underlying lesion, which led to the thrombosis.

TEST OF CHOICE
- Ultrasound for preoperative planning, augmented by venography.
- Venography/fistulography for continued evaluation and intervention to maintain patency.

BIBLIOGRAPHY
http://www.kidney.org/professionals/kdoqi/guidelines.cfm
NKF-K/DOQI Clinical Practice Guidelines for Vascular Access: update 2000. *Am J Kidney Dis.* 2001;37:S137-S181.

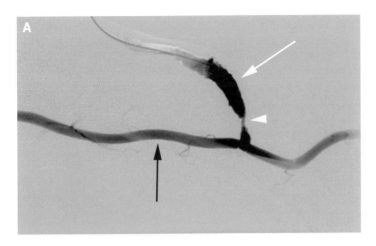

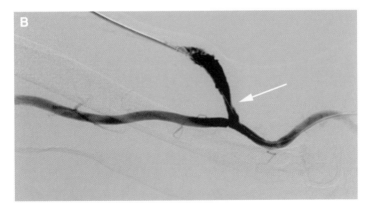

Figure 8-10 (A) Fistulogram identifies a high grade stenosis (arrowhead) adjacent to the arteriovenous anastamosis of a fistula created between the brachial artery (black arrow) and the cephalic vein (white arrow). (B) Follow up fistulogram after angioplasty reveals near complete resolution of the previously identified stenosis.

8-11. Abdominal Aortic Aneurysm

CASE HISTORY
A 55-year-old presents with pulsatile abdominal mass.

BACKGROUND
Abdominal aortic aneurysm (AAA) is caused by a degenerative process in the abdominal aorta. It is a common condition, with a prevalence of 1%–4% in the over 50 population. Aortic aneurysms are usually asymptomatic. Although the most common physical finding is a pulsatile abdominal mass, physical examination has poor predictive value in the detection of AAA. Abdominal aneurysms are not palpable in large patients, while normal aortas in thin subjects can simulate a pulsatile mass. If untreated, aneurysms gradually enlarge and eventually rupture. This can occur suddenly and carries a mortality of 80%–94%. Fifty percent of patients with ruptured aorta do not reach the hospital alive. The larger the aneurysm, the greater the risk of rupture. Rupture can be prevented by early detection of the aneurysm and endovascular repair.

TEST RATIONALE
The test of choice for detection or exclusion of AAA is sonography. It is quick, accurate, and easily performed at the bedside. Ultrasound can determine the size and extent of an aneurysm, and the presence of intraluminal thrombus (see Fig. 8-11). It is particularly useful in following the size of an aneurysm over time. Ultrasound is insensitive for detection of rupture, and unenhanced CT should be performed in the unstable patient. Contrast-enhanced CT is usually required before endograft or open repair is performed.

TEST OF CHOICE
Ultrasound of the aorta.

BIBLIOGRAPHY
Bluth E, LoCascio L. Ultrasound evaluation of the abdominal aorta. *Echocardiography*. 1996 Mar;13(2):197-206.
Brown PM, Zelt DT, Sobolev B. The risk of rupture in untreated aneurysms: the impact of size, gender, and expansion rate. *J Vasc Surg*. 2003 Feb;37(2):280-284.

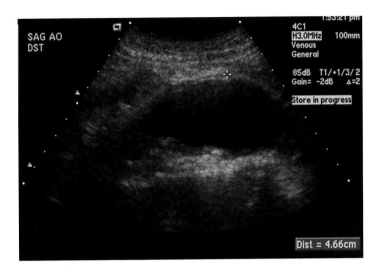

Figure 8-11 Long-axis ultrasound image of the mid-abdomen shows a dilated tubular black structure, the aorta, with maximal diameter delineated by calipers. In general, a width of more than 3 cm of the abdominal aorta indicates aneurysmal dilation.

9

IMAGING OF PEDIATRIC PATIENTS

*Sarah D. Bixby and
Carlo Buonomo*

9-1. Midgut Volvulus

CASE HISTORY
A 2-day-old, previously healthy, full-term infant presents with bilious emesis.

BACKGROUND
Intestinal malrotation occurs secondary to an embryologic defect in the normal rotation of the bowel. As early as the fifth week of gestation, the intestines, which originally form outside the embryo, begin to herniate into the umbilical cord. Ultimately the intestines will make a 270 degree rotation as they enter the abdominal cavity. An arrest in development may occur at any stage of this process, resulting in malrotated, malfixated bowel loops that are prone to volvulus. Bilious emesis is a common presenting symptom in newborn infants with malrotation and midgut volvulus. While bilious emesis may also be a symptom of any cause of intestinal obstruction, midgut volvulus is a life-threatening condition that requires emergent diagnosis. Other complications of delayed diagnosis and treatment include intestinal perforation and sepsis. A benign clinical examination should not preclude imaging evaluation in these infants who may decompensate very suddenly.

TEST RATIONALE
Plain abdominal radiographs are routinely obtained in the initial imaging of an infant with bilious emesis to evaluate for signs of bowel obstruction. The most common radiographic finding in an infant with malrotation is a normal bowel gas pattern. In some patients the stomach and proximal duodenum will appear dilated (see Fig. 9-1A). The study of choice for the diagnosis of malrotation with midgut volvulus is the upper gastrointestinal (UGI) series. It is important to be aware that infants with several or many dilated loops of bowel on plain radiographs are more likely to have a lower intestinal obstruction than midgut volvulus, and these infants are best evaluated by contrast enema before UGI. The purpose of the UGI is to identify the location of the ligament of Treitz, from the position of which we infer the degree of rotation of the remainder of the bowel. While the ligament of Treitz is not visible at UGI, its position can be deduced by the location of the duodenojejunal junction (DJJ). In a normal infant the duodenum follows a characteristic "C-loop," which places the DJJ to the left of midline at the level of the pylorus. When the intestine is malrotated, the DJJ is positioned more inferiorly and/or more midline than usual (see Fig. 9-1B). This also allows the contrast to be followed into the cecum with

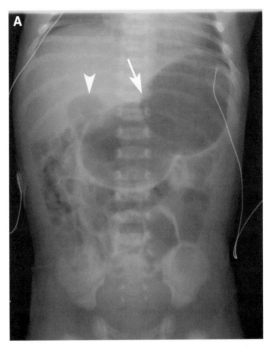

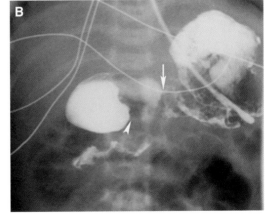

Figure 9-1 (A) AP radiograph of the abdomen in a 2-day-old infant demonstrates a dilated stomach (arrow) as well as dilatation of the proximal portion of the duodenum (arrowhead). The remainder of the bowel gas pattern is normal. (B) AP fluoroscopic spot image from an upper gastrointestinal series on the same infant. Contrast opacifies the stomach, demonstrating a nasogastric tube in place. The pylorus is indicated by the arrow. There is an abrupt tapering at the junction of the second and third portions of the duodenum (arrowhead). A small trickle of contrast outlines the third and fourth portions of the duodenum, which course into the right side of the abdomen and head inferiorly. The patient was taken directly to surgery where a midgut volvulus was reduced. AP, antereoposterior.

serial radiographs. If the cecum is in a location other than the right lower quadrant, the child is malrotated. When midgut volvulus is present there is often an abrupt tapering of the caliber of the duodenum at the site of volvulus (see Fig. 9-1B). If contrast is able to pass distal to this transition point the bowel often assumes a "corkscrew" configuration, which is diagnostic of midgut volvulus. The treatment for midgut volvulus is Ladd's procedure, which consists of untwisting the volvulus, lysis of Ladd's bands, appendectomy, and placement of the bowel back in the abdomen usually with the small bowel on the left, colon on the right.

TEST OF CHOICE
UGI series.

BIBLIOGRAPHY

Applegate KE, Anderson JM, Klatte EC. Intestinal malrotation in children: a problem-solving approach to the upper gastrointestinal series. *Radiographics*. 2006;26(5):1485-1500.

Ortiz-Neira CL. The corkscrew sign: midgut volvulus. *Radiology*. 2007;242(1):315-316.

9-2. Croup

CASE HISTORY
A 5-month-old male with stridor is brought in to the emergency room.

BACKGROUND
Croup is a common illness in young children. Viral agents, most commonly the parainfluenza viruses, are responsible for the majority of cases of croup. Croup affects children between 1 and 6 years of age, and most cases occur in late fall and winter seasons. Croup is usually a self-limited disease with little morbidity, though in rare instances complications may ensue. Few children require hospitalization to manage acute, life-threatening respiratory compromise, though most infants are well-enough to be managed at home. In many cases the symptoms are alleviated by humidification of the air (such as a steam bath) or a few minutes of breathing cool, night air. It is important to differentiate croup, a relatively benign disease process, from other more sinister causes of airway obstruction, such as epiglottitis or foreign body aspiration. Patients with epiglottitis are usually ill-appearing and hold their neck in a characteristic "sniffing" position to facilitate breathing. In cases of foreign body aspiration the symptoms tend to begin acutely, and the caretakers often are aware of the potentially aspirated object. In contrast to these conditions, children with croup experience symptoms of an upper respiratory infection, which then progresses to a "barking" cough and inspiratory stridor.

TEST RATIONALE
Although croup causes diffuse inflammation and edema of the entire upper airway, on radiographs of the airway croup is manifested as predominantly subglottic narrowing. The subglottic airway is the narrowest part of a child's airway, and therefore the effects of the airway swelling are most pronounced in this area. Anteroposterior (AP) radiographs reveal gradual tapering of the subglottic airway, resulting in the "steeple" sign (see Figs. 9-2A and 9-2B). In some cases the hypopharynx will be hyperextended with air. The lateral radiograph of the neck is less helpful than the AP view, as the subglottic narrowing is more difficult to appreciate in this projection. The lateral view does play a valuable role in differentiating croup from other conditions that are better evaluated in this projection, such as epiglottitis (manifested as a thickened, enlarged epiglottitis), retropharyngeal abscess (abnormal thickening of the retropharyngeal soft tissues), or adenoidal and tonsillar hypertrophy. Despite the characteristic imaging

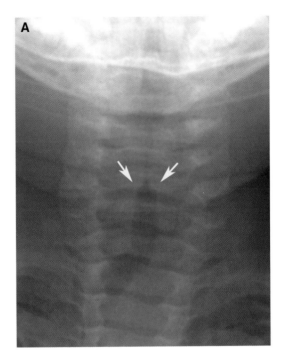

Figure 9-2 (A) AP view of the neck and upper airway in a 9-month-old normal infant demonstrates the normal appearance of the subglottic airway, with an abrupt "shouldering" of the airway just below the level of the vocal folds (arrows). Incidental note is made of right lateral buckling of the intrathoracic trachea secondary to the phase of inspiration. (B) AP view of the neck and upper airway in a 5-month-old male with stridor demonstrates gradual tapering of the subglottic airway with loss of the normal "shouldering" normal seen in this region (arrows) yielding the classic "steeple" sign. This child was diagnosed with croup. AP, antereoposterior.

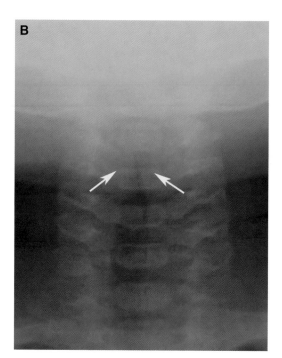

Figure 9-2   Continued.

features, radiographs should not be relied upon for definitive diagnosis of croup, as in approximately 50% of cases there will be no imaging findings to suggest the diagnosis. In the appropriate clinical setting, "negative" radiographs should not exclude the diagnosis of croup.

TEST OF CHOICE
AP and lateral radiographs of the neck.

BIBLIOGRAPHY
Bjornson CL, Johnson DW. Croup. *Lancet.* 2008;371(9609):329-339.
John SD, Swischuk LE. Stridor and upper airway obstruction in infants and children. *Radiographics.* 1992;12(4):625-643.

9-3. Langerhans Cell Histiocytosis

CASE HISTORY
A 21-month-old male presents with pain and swelling in the right thigh.

BACKGROUND
Langerhans cell histiocytosis (LCH) encompasses a spectrum of disorders ranging from a solitary bone lesion to disseminated multiorgan disease. Most children with LCH (~70%) have a localized osseous lesion and present with symptoms of pain and tenderness at the site of the lesion, low-grade fever, elevated erythrocyte sedimentation rate, and/or peripheral eosinophilia. Children with LCH are usually younger than 15 years of age. While the skull is the most frequent site of involvement, LCH may involve nearly any bone, with a predilection toward flat bones. The presence of both aggressive and nonaggressive imaging features is typical for LCH. Eosinophilic granuloma (EG), Hand-Schuller–Christian disease, and Letterer–Siwe disease are terms previously employed to describe specific manifestations of LCH ranging from localized (EG) to fulminant, disseminated disease (Letterer–Siwe). Today LCH is considered a continuum of a disease rather than discrete, individual entities. Interestingly, some lesions spontaneously resolve without treatment. For osseous lesions which do not resolve, treatment consists of curettage and bone grafting. Lesions rarely recur.

TEST RATIONALE
The most common form of LCH, the localized osseous lesion, is most often detected on plain radiographs obtained for evaluation of musculoskeletal pain or tenderness (see Figs. 9-3A and 9-3B). Radiographs remain the most valuable imaging means of detecting and characterizing these lesions. The correct diagnosis is often suggested on the basis of the plain radiographic features even when newer, more sophisticated imaging has been performed (such as computed tomography [CT] or magnetic resonance imaging [MRI]). The imaging features of LCH vary depending on the location of the lesions. Lesions within the long bones often have an aggressive appearance manifested by endosteal scalloping, cortical thinning, and permeative bone destruction. Such lesions mimic other processes such as osteomyelitis, and malignant neoplasms, such as Ewing sarcoma, lymphoma, leukemia, and metastasis. In the spine, LCH causes a characteristic vertebra plana deformity with near-total loss of vertebral body height. In the skull, LCH has a more benign imaging appearance, often with sharp borders that give

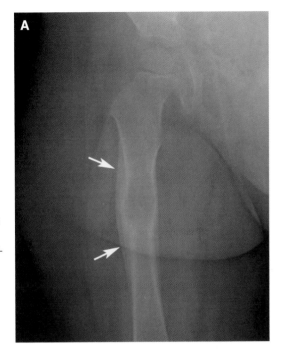

Figure 9-3   (A) AP radiograph of the femur in a 21-month-old male with a known diagnosis of LCH demonstrates an ill-defined, lucent lesion within the proximal femoral diaphysis with endosteal scalloping, and smooth periosteal new bone formation (arrows). (B) Lateral radiograph of the femur in the same 21-month-old infant once again demonstrates an ill-defined, lucent, diaphyseal lesion with smooth periosteal new bone formation (arrows). AP, antereoposterior; LCH, Langerhans cell histiocytosis.

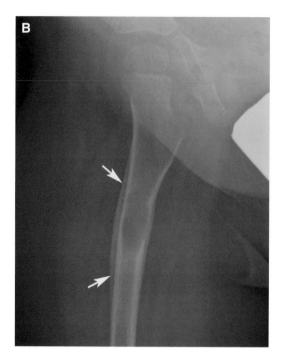

Figure 9-3 Continued.

the lesion a "punched out" or beveled appearance. In some cases, a sequestrum is present, as well as an accompanying soft tissue mass.

CT is unnecessary in the work-up of LCH, though CT may be helpful in evaluating the degree of cortical destruction in patients deemed at high fracture risk. CT does have a role in guiding biopsy of suspicious lesions. MRI is preferred over CT for initial diagnostic evaluation secondary to its superior ability to detect bone marrow involvement and delineate associated soft tissue masses without the use of ionizing radiation.

TEST OF CHOICE
Plain radiographs.

BIBLIOGRAPHY
Azouz EM, Saigal G, Rodriguez MM, et al. Langerhans' cell histiocytosis: pathology, imaging and treatment of skeletal involvement. *Pediatr Radiol.* 2005;35:103-115.
Hoover KB, Rosenthal DI, Mankin H. Langerhans cell histiocytosis. *Skeletal Radiol.* 2007;36:95-104.

9-4. Intussusception

CASE HISTORY
A 3-month-old female with inconsolability and currant jelly stools is brought in to the emergency room.

BACKGROUND
Intussusception is a term used to describe the invagination of one bowel loop into a more distal segment, usually occurring at the ileocolic junction. It is the most common cause of acute bowel obstruction in infants, and most often affects children between the ages of 5 months and 3 years. Nearly all (95%) cases of intussusception in infants are considered idiopathic and likely related to enlarged mesenteric lymph nodes. Symptoms include intermittent abdominal pain, vomiting, and right upper quadrant mass. When rectal bleeding is also present, the diagnosis of intussusception is almost certain. Imaging studies are an important part of the diagnostic evaluation, as prompt diagnosis and treatment is critical to avoid bowel infarction and perforation.

TEST RATIONALE
Plain radiographs are imperative in the initial imaging evaluation of a child with concern for intussusception. Classic radiographic signs of intussusception include the "crescent" or "meniscus" sign which describe the appearance of the intussusceptum (the intussuscepted segment) outlined by gas in the intussuscepiens (the receiving segment) (see Fig. 9-4A). The "target" sign describes the appearance of an intussusception oriented parallel to the x-ray beam, as the mesenteric fat centrally within the intussusception appears lower in attenuation than the surrounding bowel wall. Absence of stool or gas in the cecum is suggestive of intussusception, though this is not diagnostic and should be interpreted in context with the patient's clinical presentation. In a child with high clinical suspicion for intussusception the lack of bowel gas in the right lower quadrant is a concerning finding, especially when there is bowel gas elsewhere in the abdomen. Radiographs also assess for free intraperitoneal air, a sign of bowel perforation.

In patients in whom the diagnosis of intussusception is uncertain based on clinical or radiographic grounds, ultrasound (US) is the next preferred imaging modality (Fig. 9-4B). In experienced hands US is able to detect intussusception in up to 100% of cases. Intussusception has a characteristic appearance at US. In tranverse plane the alternating hyper- and hypo-echoic layers of the bowel wall assume a "target" appearance. Doppler US is helpful in demonstrating the presence of blood flow within the bowel wall.

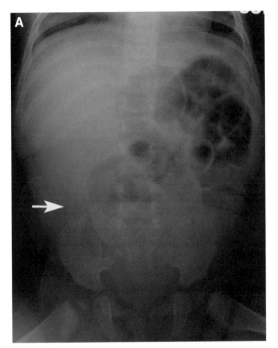

Figure 9-4   (A) AP supine radiograph of the abdomen in a 3-month-old female demonstrates multiple dilated loops of bowel occupying the left side of the abdomen. There is a paucity of gas in the right abdomen (arrow), and a gas-filled cecum is not identified. (B) Transverse ultrasound image of the right lower quadrant in the same 3-month-old female demonstrates a round mass with alternating hypo- and hyper-echoic layers (arrow), giving the mass a "target" appearance. AP, antereoposterior.

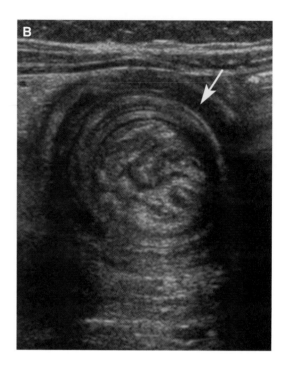

Figure 9-4   Continued.

Air enema is the treatment of choice for reduction of ileocolic intussusception. The intussusceptum is monitored under fluoroscopy as it is reduced back through the ileocecal valve by air insufflated into the rectum under pressure. The pressure is constantly monitored so as to avoid the risk of causing bowel perforation. Pediatric surgeons are made aware of an ongoing enema reduction in case of perforation which would necessitate an urgent operation, though this occurs in less than 2% of cases. Air enema is effective at reducing ileocolic intussusception in greater than 85% of cases. Surgery is performed in the case of an unsuccessful air reduction.

TEST OF CHOICE
Abdominal radiographs +/– US.

BIBLIOGRAPHY
Daneman A, Navarro O. Intussusception part 1: a review of diagnostic approaches. *Pediatr Radiol.* 2003;33:79-85.
Ko HS, Schenk JP, Tröger J et al. Current radiological management of intussusception in children. *Eur Radiol.* 2007;17(9):2411-2421.

9-5. Slipped Capital Femoral Epiphysis

CASE HISTORY
A 15-year-old male presents with left hip pain and limp.

BACKGROUND
Slipped capital femoral epiphysis (SCFE) is the most common causes of hip pain in adolescents. SCFE represents an atraumatic fracture through the proximal femoral physis, which results in displacement of the femoral epiphysis. SCFE occurs in children between the ages of 8 and 17 years, and boys are affected more frequently than girls. The slip usually occurs during a growth spurt when the proximal femoral physis is at its widest and oriented rather obliquely. Risk factors include malnutrition, endocrine abnormalities, and prior developmental dysplasia of the hip. The disease has a higher incidence in black children and in children who are overweight. Slips are bilateral in 30%–37% of cases. Treatment consists of placement of a screw or pin across the femoral physis to stabilize the femoral head. Reduction of the femoral head is not performed before pinning, as this may increase the risk of avascular necrosis of the femoral head.

TEST RATIONALE
AP and lateral radiographs of the hips are diagnostic of SCFE in nearly all cases. The femoral head on the affected side is displaced posteromedially with respect to the femoral neck (see Fig. 9-5A). In early or mild cases, this finding may only be appreciated on the lateral view . When the findings are subtle it is helpful to draw a line along the superior aspect of the femoral neck on the AP radiograph called Klein's line. In normal patients, Klein's line will pass through approximately 20% of the femoral head. In SCFE Klein's line will not intersect the femoral head, or will intersect only a very small fraction (<20%). Associated findings on radiographs include apparent widening of the physis on the affected side and relative demineralization of the ipsilateral hip (see Fig. 9-5B). The metaphyseal blanch sign is another imaging feature of SCFE that refers to the increased sclerosis in the proximal femoral metaphysis of the affected hip. This sclerosis most likely represents a healing response to the SCFE. On the basis of radiographs SCFE is classified as mild, moderate, or severe. This grading system assesses the degree of displacement of the femoral head with respect to the width of the femoral metaphyis. The metaphysis is divided into thirds; mild, moderate, and severe slips are defined femoral head displacement of 1/3, 2/3, or the full width of the metaphysis, respectively.

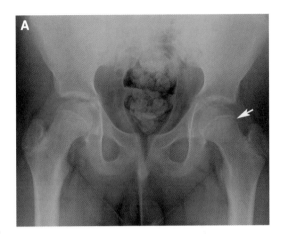

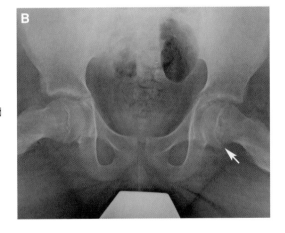

Figure 9-5   (A) AP radiograph of the hips in a 15-year-old male demonstrates mild osteopenia of the left hip. There is widening of the femoral physis on the left side (arrow). The right hip is normal. (B) Frog-leg lateral view of bilateral hips in the same 15-year-old patient demonstrates mild posteromedial displacement of the left femoral head, associated with widening of the proximal physis (arrow). The right hip is normal.
AP, antereoposterior.

MRI is a useful adjunct in equivocal cases, or when a "pre-slip" is suspected. When a "pre-slip" is present, patients often complain of hip pain and weakness. Radiographs demonstrate no displacement of the femoral head, though physeal abnormalities are present, which herald an impending slip. While these subtle changes may be appreciable on radiographs, MRI is much more sensitive for detecting the physeal widening and osteopenia that occurs at this stage.

TEST OF CHOICE
AP and lateral radiographs of the hips.

BIBLIOGRAPHY
Boles CA, El-Khoury GY. Slipped capital femoral epiphysis. *Radiographics*. 1997;17:809-823.
Umans H, Liebling MS, Moy L, et al. Slipped capital femoral epiphysis: a physeal lesion diagnosed by MRI, with radiographic and CT correlation. *Skeletal Radiol*. 1998;27:139-144.

9-6. Neuroblastoma

CASE HISTORY
A 23-month-old male presents with diarrhea and flank mass.

BACKGROUND
Neuroblastoma is a malignant childhood neoplasm, which is often challenging to diagnose because of its myriad imaging appearances and multiple potential organs of involvement. Neuroblastoma is the third most common pediatric malignancy (after leukemia and central nervous system [CNS] tumors) and the second most common abdominal neoplasm in children (after Wilms tumor). Most children with neuroblastoma are between 1 and 5 years in age. Patients often present with nonspecific constitutional symptoms which mimic a viral illness. Other symptoms are related to mass effect and depend upon tumor location (for example, hypertension, urinary frequency, dyspnea). Neuroblastoma may present as an abdominal, pelvic, thoracic, or cervical mass. The presence of bone pain suggests metastatic osseous involvement. The International Neuroblastoma Staging System (INSS) categorizes the disease into four stages depending upon the resectability of the tumor and the presence of metastatic spread. Age and stage at diagnosis are the most important predictors of survival.

TEST RATIONALE
Imaging recommendations are directed by symptoms, which vary greatly from patient to patient. Plain radiographs demonstrate a soft tissue mass only if it is causing significant displacement of organs or eroding into adjacent vertebral bodies. A mass large enough to be noticed on radiographs may already be palpable at physical examination. US is much more helpful in detecting small abdominal or pelvic masses which escape physical detection (see Fig. 9-6A). The adrenal glands are the most common site of involvement of neuroblastoma, a location difficult to palpate but easily evaluated with US. At US the mass will appear to glide past adjacent abdominal organs with respiratory movement unless those organs are also involved with the tumor. This imaging feature is unique to US and allows improved clarification of the organ of origin. A classic imaging feature of neuroblastoma is the encasement of blood vessels rather than displacement.

CT and MRI are useful as a supplement to US to provide detailed anatomic information for presurgical planning and staging (see Fig. 9-6B). Nearly all abdominal neuroblastomas demonstrate calcification on CT. The mass appears lobular and without a discrete capsule may invade the psoas muscle or neural foramina. Lymph nodes, when present, may blend

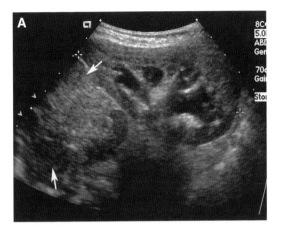

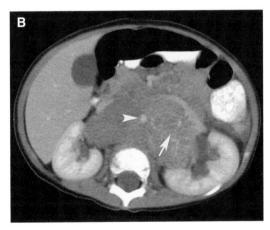

Figure 9-6 (A) Longitudinal US image of the left kidney in a 23-month-old boy demonstrates a large, heterogeneous suprarenal mass (arrows) with focal punctate areas of increased echogenicity likely representing calcification. There is mild dilatation of the left renal collecting system. (B) Axial image from a contrast-enhanced CT of the abdomen and pelvis in the same 23-month-old male demonstrates a large, suprarenal, retroperitoneal mass, which contains multiple punctate calcifications (arrow). The mass is encasing the aorta (arrowhead). Although the kidneys appear normal, the left kidney is displaced inferiorly by the mass.

CT, computed tomography; US, ultrasound.

into the primary mass and be indistinguishable from it. When the diagnosis has been established (usually on the basis of biopsy), patients are evaluated with bone scan to assess for sites of skeletal involvement, as well as a meta-iodobenzylguanidine (MIBG) scan to assess for metastatic disease.

TEST OF CHOICE
Abdominal US.

BIBLIOGRAPHY
Hiorns MP, Owens CM. Radiology of neuroblastoma in children. *Eur Radiol.* 2001;11:2071-2081.
Papaioannou G and McHugh K. Neuroblastoma in childhood: review and radiological findings. *Cancer Imaging.* 2005;5:116-127.

9-7. Pyloric Stenosis

CASE HISTORY
A 5-week-old female presents with progressive, forceful vomiting after every feed.

BACKGROUND
Infants with pyloric stenosis are normal at birth and develop forceful, non-bilious vomiting in the first few weeks of life. The vomiting is typically described as "projectile" in quality. As the condition progresses the vomiting becomes more and more frequent, and the infant may become dehydrated and malnourished. The disease is caused by abnormal thickening and rigidity of the pyloric channel, which leads to gastric outlet obstruction. The etiology of the disease is not well understood. Pyloric stenosis is a relatively common disease, and occurs more frequently in boys than in girls (4:1). Infants are typically between 3 and 6 weeks of age at presentation. Definitive treatment is a pyloromyotomy.

TEST RATIONALE
While vomiting is a common symptom in early infancy, patients with pyloric stenosis have a characteristic age and clinical presentation. Although a palpable "olive" is a hallmark of the disease, this usually requires an experienced surgeon and a quiet, relaxed infant. A more reliable means of obtaining a definitive diagnosis before surgery is US evaluation of the pylorus. A normal pylorus is a nearly imperceptible ring of tissue, which actively peristalses to allow the passage of gastric contents into the duodenum. Under real-time imaging it is usually possible to identify a normal pylorus while watching the stomach empty. When the stomach is markedly distended the pylorus may be displaced posteriorly and will therefore be difficult to visualize sonographically. In some instances it may be helpful to decompress the stomach with a nasogastric tube, or repeat the examination after several hours to allow the stomach adequate time to empty. In patients with pyloric stenosis the pylorus appears markedly thickened and elongated. While measurements vary by institution, a pyloric muscle thickness greater than 3.0 mm on one side of the channel is considered diagnostic of pyloric stenosis. This measurement is most accurately obtained on a longitudinal image through the channel (see Fig. 9-7). While channel length tends to be increased in patients with pyloric stenosis (that is, nearly always greater than 15 mm) the length of the pyloric channel is not as indicative of pyloric stenosis as muscle thickness. In pyloric stenosis the pyloric channel

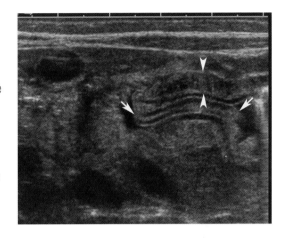

Figure 9-7
Longitudinal image through the pylorus in the same infant with pyloric stenosis with arrows denoting the length of the pyloric channel, and arrowheads denoting where to measure pyloric muscle thickness (which measured 4 mm in this infant).

remains fixed over the period of the examination and little to no fluid will pass through the channel into the duodenum. In challenging cases it is helpful to feed the infant sugar water and acquire images with the infant in a right lateral oblique position to best allow fluid to enter the antrum and outline the pylorus.

TEST OF CHOICE
Pyloric US.

BIBLIOGRAPHY

Hernanz-Schulman, M. Infantile hypertrophic pyloric stenosis. *Radiology.* 2003;227:319-331.

Teele RL, Smith EH. Ultrasound in the diagnosis of idiopathic hypertrophic pyloric stenosis. *N Engl J Med.* 1977;296(20):1149-1150.

9-8. Posterior Urethral Valves

CASE HISTORY
A 5-week-old male with history of prenatal hydronephrosis presents for evaluation of the urinary tract.

BACKGROUND
Posterior urethral valves (PUVs) occur exclusively in the male urethra. The valves consist of a thin membrane within the posterior urethra, which may be complete or incomplete, thereby causing various degrees of urinary obstruction and renal insufficiency. Male infants with complete PUVs are unable to void, prompting a diagnostic work-up shortly after birth. More commonly infants are diagnosed with PUVs prenatally based on an abnormal-screening US examination. Urethral obstruction in the neonatal period is nearly always secondary to PUVs. In cases of incomplete PUVs the diagnosis may escape detection for years. These patients may present at a later age with a history of repeated urinary tract infections, failure to thrive, voiding dysfunction, or unexplained renal failure.

TEST RATIONALE
Renal ultrasound (RUS) is indicated in any newborn male who fails to pass urine within 24 hours of birth, and any infant with a history of prenatal hydronephrosis. In the first scenario the US is performed semiurgently, whereas in the latter scenario the study is performed approximately 1 week after birth, as most neonates are naturally dehydrated in the first few days of life which may cause falsely reassuring findings on US. RUS assesses for signs of urinary tract obstruction, such as hydronephrosis, hydroureter, and an enlarged and thickened bladder (see Fig. 9-8A). The dilated, posterior urethra is often identified with a classic "keyhole" configuration (See Fig. 9-8B). Renal dysplasia should be suspected if the kidney appears small, echogenic, and with cortical cysts. In severe cases urinoma or urinary ascites may be present. The sonographic findings of PUVs are similar to other conditions such as "prune belly syndrome," and "megacystis-microcolon-intestinal hypoperistalsis syndrome." These entities can readily be differentiated from one another based on the other clinical features and findings at voiding cystourethrogram (VCUG).

VCUG is performed in combination with RUS to confirm the diagnosis of PUVs and to assess for vesicoureteral reflux. During voiding the posterior urethera appears dilated with an abrupt transition at the level of the valves to a narrow anterior urethra. The valve cusps may be identified

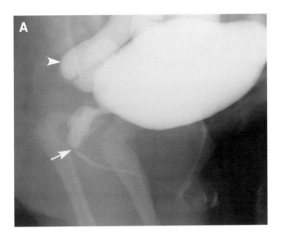

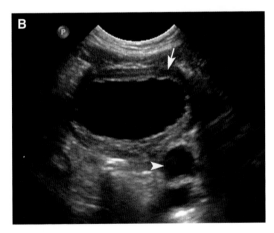

Figure 9-8   (A) Lateral fluoroscopic spot image of the urethra in a 5-week-old male with history of prenatal hydronephrosis demonstrated dilatation of the posterior urethra, with an abrupt change of caliber to a narrow anterior urethra with evidence of posterior urethral valves at the site of caliber change (arrow). The bladder capacity is large, and unilateral vesicoureteral reflux is present (arrowhead). (B) Transverse US image of the bladder in the same patient demonstrates circumferential bladder wall thickening (arrow). The left distal ureter is dilated (arrowhead).

US, ultrasound.

during the voiding phase of a VCUG if they are outlined by contrast. The verumontanum appears enlarged. The urinary bladder commonly has a large capacity, and the bladder wall is trabeculated, with multiple saccules, and diverticulae. Vesicoureteral reflux may be unilateral, bilateral, or completely absent.

While valuable for the anatomic information they provide, RUS and VCUG do not provide information regarding the functional status of the kidneys, which will ultimately be important in determining the degree of renal insufficiency.

TEST OF CHOICE
US+VCUG.

BIBLIOGRAPHY
Gilsanz V, Miller JH, Reid BS. Ultrasonic characteristics of posterior urethral valves. *Radiology.* 1982;145(1):143-145.
Macpherson RI, Leithiser RE, Gordon L, Turner WR. Posterior urethral valves: an update and review. *Radiographics.* 1986;6(5):753-791.

9-9. Congenital Cystic Adenomatoid Malformation

CASE HISTORY
Asymptomatic newborn male infant with prenatally diagnosed lung mass presents for further evaluation of the lungs.

BACKGROUND
With ongoing advances in prenatal imaging an increasing number of conditions are being diagnosed in utero, including congenital cystic adenomatoid malformation (CCAM). CCAM is a relatively rare lesion, which results from an arrest in normal lung development. Males and females are affected equally. Small lesions may be entirely asymptomatic, while larger masses may lead to fetal hydrops, polyhydramnios, or even intrauterine fetal demise. Most lesions involve only one lobe. CCAMs have been demonstrated to regress antenatally. This has important implications for prenatal counseling given that the prognosis for the fetus often depends on the size of the mass. The differential diagnosis includes congenital diaphragmatic hernia and pulmonary sequestration. According to the Stocker classification there are three main types of CCAM. Type1 lesions consist of a single or several large cysts (>3 cm). Type 1 lesions are the most frequent type of CCAM and are associated with the best prognosis. Type 2 lesions are composed of multiple medium-sized cysts (<2 cm). Type 3 lesions consist of innumerable tiny cysts, and are associated with the worst prognosis. Definitive treatment is surgical resections. Even asymptomatic lesions are resected in light of the risk of future infection or malignant degeneration of the lesion, although this occurs rarely.

TEST RATIONALE
The prenatal imaging of CCAM relies heavily on US. The US appearance of CCAM is an echogenic mass in the thorax, which may cause displacement of the heart and mediastinal structures depending upon its size. In the newborn period chest radiographs and computed tomography are the diagnostic imaging modalities of choice (see Fig. 9-9A). On plain radiographs CCAM appears as multiple air- or fluid-filled cystic structures, which cause displacement of the heart and mediastinum. Unfortunately, not all CCAMs are large enough to be detectable on a plain radiograph. For any infant with an abnormal chest radiograph (that is, presence of a mass) or an infant with a normal chest radiograph but high clinical suspicion (that is, mass noted on prenatal US) a contrast-enhanced CT of the thorax is indicated (see

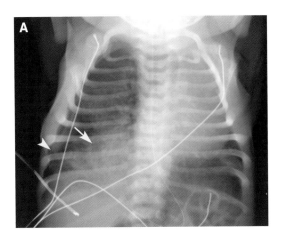

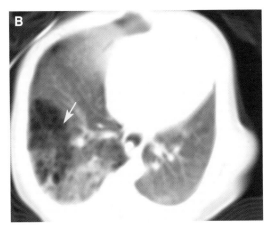

Figure 9-9 (A) AP radiograph of the chest in a newborn infant with a suspected lung mass based on prenatal ultrasound demonstrates a large mass in the right lower lobe (arrow), which is causing shift of the heart and mediastinum into the left chest. There is also a small right pneumothorax (arrowhead). (B) Axial image from a contrast-enhanced CT through the chest demonstrates a mass within the right lower lobe which contains multiple cystic cavities (arrow).

AP, antereoposterior; CT, computed tomography.

Fig. 9-9B). CT provides more detailed anatomic information regarding the nature of the cysts (size and number) as well as the relationship of the lesion to the surrounding lung parenchyma. The CT is performed with intravenous contrast to best evaluate for arterial feeders arising directly from the descending aorta, which would suggest pulmonary sequestration rather than a strict CCAM, although there are hybrid lesions in which CCAM and sequestration coexist.

TEST OF CHOICE
US of the chest.

BIBLIOGRAPHY
Adzick NS, Harrison MR, Crombleholme TM, et al. Fetal lung lesions: management and outcome. *Am J Obstet Gynecol.* 1998;179(4):884-889.

Calvert JK, Lakhoo K. Antenatally suspected congenital cystic adenomatoid malformation of the lung: postnatal investigation and timing of surgery. *J Pediatr Surg.* 2007;42:411-414.

9-10. Ewing Sarcoma

CASE HISTORY
A 4-year-old male complains of left leg pain and walks with a limp.

BACKGROUND
Ewing sarcoma is the second most common primary malignant bone tumor in childhood (behind osteosarcoma). Ewing sarcoma is one of the small, round, blue cell tumors in the same family as neuroblastoma, rhabdomyosarcoma, and non-Hodgkin's lymphoma. The tumor cells contain a characteristic genetic translocation also expressed by primitive neuroectodermal tumors (PNET). Males and females are affected equally, and lesions are most commonly discovered in the second decade of life. The lower extremity and pelvis are the most commonly affected sites of involvement. Patients usually present with complaints of musculoskeletal pain, often described as chronic and unrelenting in nature. A palpable mass is appreciated in some cases. Systemic signs and symptoms such as weight loss, fever, and elevated erythrocyte sedimentation rate may also be present. Treatment consists of systemic chemotherapy, local radiation therapy, and surgical resection. The type of surgery depends on tumor site and extent, and limb-salvage surgeries are clearly preferred over amputation when at all possible.

TEST RATIONALE
Evaluation of a child with pain referable to a bone or joint begins with plain radiographs. Ewing sarcoma of the long bones is commonly middiaphyseal or metadiaphyseal. A lesion involving a flat bone, such as the iliac wing or scapula, is also characteristic of Ewing sarcoma. Ewing sarcoma is characteristically lytic, though there may be a mixed lytic/blastic appearance (Fig. 9-10A). Associated periosteal new bone formation is present in nearly all cases and is classically described as having an "onion-skinning" or "hair on end" appearance (Fig. 9-10B). A soft tissue mass usually present, which is best evaluated with cross-section imaging methods. Radiographic features of Ewings sarcoma are often very similar to Langerhans cell histiocytosis (LCH), osteomyelitis, and osteosarcoma.

   MRI is the preferred imaging modality for further evaluation of radiographically aggressive-appearing osseous lesions. MRI depicts the extent of the primary lesion as well as assesses for skip lesions. Relative to the adjacent bone marrow Ewing sarcoma is low-signal on T1-weighted images and bright on T2-weighted images.

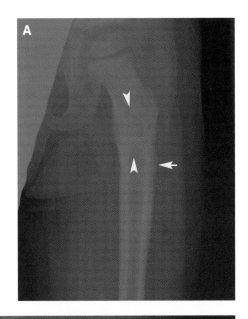

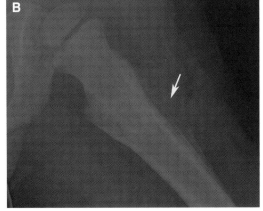

Figure 9-10 (A) AP radiograph of the left femur demonstrates a mixed lytic/sclerotic lesion (arrowheads) within the proximal femoral diaphysis with a permeative pattern of bone destruction, ill-defined margins, and discontinuous periosteal elevation (arrow). (B) Lateral radiograph of the femur in the same 4-year-old boy demonstrates to better advantage the subtle "sunburst" pattern to the periosteal new bone formation (arrow). There is also mild displacement of the overlying soft tissue planes suggesting mass effect.

AP, antereoposterior.

All patients diagnosed with Ewing sarcoma ultimately undergo CT of the chest to assess for lung metastases. Once the diagnosis has been established a complete work-up also includes bone scan to detect skip lesions in the bone of the primary tumor and metastatic or synchronous lesions. After treatment most patients are followed with MRI of the primary tumor site, chest CT, and bone scan to evaluate for tumor recurrence and metastatic spread.

TEST OF CHOICE
Plain radiographs.

BIBLIOGRAPHY
Meyer JS, Mackenzie W. Malignant bone tumors and limb-salvage surgery in children. *Pediatr Radiol.* 2004;34(8):606-613.
Yaw KM. Pediatric bone tumors. *Semin Surg Oncol.* 1999;16(2):173-183.

A PRIMER ON THE USE OF NUCLEAR MEDICINE TESTS

Amir H. Khandani

PET overview

BRIEF OVERVIEW OF FDG PET

The radioisotope portion of the molecules used in positron emission tomography (PET) imaging emits two photons that travel at the speed of light in exactly opposite directions (180 degrees apart). Coincident detection of these two photons by oppositely-positioned detectors in the PET scanner results in images with a much higher resolution compared to the conventional, single photon nuclear medicine studies, and produces the possibility of quantitative measurement of the tracer uptake in a lesion of interest by measuring standard uptake value (SUV). In PET computed tomography (CT), the patient undergoes a CT scan, followed by a PET scan without changing the patient position. PET-CT allows the fusion of the metabolic information on PET with the anatomic information on CT. PET (or PET-CT) for most oncologic indications (whole-body PET) is acquired from the base of the skull through the upper thighs. In some instances, such as in melanoma patients, PET is acquired from the vertex of the skull through the toes.

Tumor imaging with 2-[^{18}F] fluoro-2-deoxy-D-glucose (FDG) is based on the principle of increased glucose metabolism of cancer cells. FDG is identical to glucose with the only difference that one of the hydroxyl groups of glucose has been replaced by radioactive fluorine. FDG is taken up by the cancer cells in the same way as glucose but since it cannot be metabolized, it is trapped in the cancer cells and constitutes the basis for tumor visualization on PET.

PATIENT PREPARATION

Patients are instructed to fast for at least 4 hours before the PET appointment. Glucose containing drinks and intravenous (IV) glucose must be avoided at least 4 hours before FDG injection as well. The fasting state lowers the serum glucose level so that FDG has less competition for uptake by the tumor. Muscle uptake is also minimized by fasting through lowering the serum insulin level. Low FDG uptake in the muscles improves the tumor to background ratio and the image quality.

High glucose level in diabetic patients can also decrease the image quality. It is well known that high glucose level decreases the tumor intensity on FDG PET and that lesions might be missed. However, while a normal glucose level in diabetic patients before FDG injection is desirable, it often cannot be achieved. Therefore, from a practical stand point, it may be reasonable to perform the scan even with a high glucose level and interpret the findings. Should the images be "diagnostic enough," and, for instance, the patient be upstaged, the low quality of images may not matter. A repeat scan should be considered, when a false-negative scan is suspected (for example, rising CA-125 in a patient with ovarian cancer, high glucose level, and negative FDG PET).

MOST COMMON INDICATIONS FOR FDG PET IN ONCOLOGY

Two general considerations (1) FDG PET is overall on a patient basis more sensitive than bone scan for bone metastases, although on a lesion basis, it may be less sensitive than bone scan in breast cancer. In any case, FDG PET should be performed first if only one imaging study is to be ordered even in breast cancer. A bone scan can be later added, if the likelihood that the patient is under-staged remains high. (2) A brain CT or magnetic resonance imaging (MRI) is needed whenever brain metastases are suspected. Due to high glucose metabolism of the brain, FDG PET may miss brain metastases.

The indications presented subsequently in the alphabetic order of various primaries are the most commonly used ones and will need regular updates. More data regarding the impact of FDG PET on disease outcome, particularly in regard to its use in therapy monitoring, will be available in the coming years.

Bladder cancer: confirm distant disease suspected on CT/MRI; assess for further disease sites and to identify the best site for biopsy

Breast cancer: staging; restaging

Cervical cancer: radiation therapy planning; restaging

Colorectal cancer: staging; restaging (rising carcinoembryonic antigen (CEA) level of unknown source)

Endometrial cancer: to confirm distant disease suspected on CT/MRI; to assess for further disease sites, and to obtain the best site for biopsy.

Esophageal cancer: staging

Gastric cancer: confirm distant disease suspected on CT/MRI; assess for further disease sites, and to identify the best site for biopsy (metastatic sites tend to be more intense than the primary site)

Head and neck cancers: assessing for primary site of disease in tumor of unknown origin; nodal staging; distant staging; radiation therapy planning; restaging

Lung cancer: assessing indeterminate lung lesion for malignancy; mediastinal staging; distant staging; radiation therapy planning; restaging

Lymphoma: staging; surveillance; restaging

Melanoma: staging, surveillance; restaging

Multiple myeloma: staging, restaging

Pancreatic cancer: confirm distant disease suspected on CT/MRI; assess for additional disease sites and to identify the best site for biopsy (metastatic sites tend to be more intense than the primary site)

Ovarian cancer: restaging (rising CA-125 of unknown source)

Renal cell cancer: confirm distant disease suspected on CT/MRI; assess for further disease sites and to identify the best site for biopsy (metastatic sites tend to be more intense than the primary site)

Sarcoma/retroperitoneal mass of unknown origin: guiding biopsy to the most intense site to obtain the highest tumor grade

Seminoma: differentiating viable tumor from scar in residual retroperitoneal mass after chemotherapy

BIBLIOGRAPHY

Khandani AH and Sheik A. Nuclear Medicine. In *Clinical Radiation Oncology*. Gunderson LL and Tepper JE. 2nd edition Philadelphia, PA: Elsevier. 207-214.

10-1. Brain Death

CASE HISTORY
An 18-year-old male with severe head injuries during a car accident, presented to the emergency department (ED) unresponsive with no gross motor function. There was loss of brain stem functions on neurologic examination, an isoelectric electroencephalogram (EEG), and positive apnea testing.

BACKGROUND
Timely diagnosis of brain death is important when organ donation is considered.

TEST RATIONALE
The diagnosis of brain death is primarily a clinical one. However, confirmatory tests can be used to increase certainty. Radionuclide brain scan is one of them). This is a noninvasive, rapid, easy-to-perform test, and an abnormal radionuclide brain scan is more specific than isoelectric EEG and almost diagnostic for brain death. Depending on the radiotracer used, only perfusion to the intracranial vessels (perfusion agents such as Technetium-99m DTPA) or perfusion, and uptake of radiotracer in the brain (Technetium-99m HMPAO) can be assessed. Lack of perfusion of the brain indicates brain death (see Fig. 10-1). The possibility of assessing the radiotracer uptake in the brain increases the level of certainty about the diagnosis, especially in the case of inadequate perfusion images. The latter tracers are increasingly used and expect to replace the perfusion-only tracers entirely. The entire study with the newer tracers requires approximately 20 minutes to complete.

TEST OF CHOICE
Radionuclide brain scan.

BIBLIOGRAPHY
Zeisman HA, O'Malley, JP, Thrall JH. *Nuclear Medicine, The Requisites*, 3rd edition. Philadelphia, PA: Elsevier. 2005:435-438.

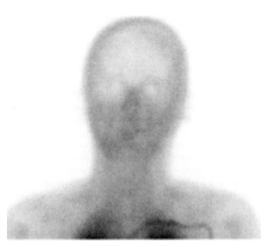

Figure 10-1   No visualization of the brain, consistent with brain death in proper clinical setting.

10-2. Cholecystitis

CASE HISTORY
A 29-year-old female presents with acute right upper quadrant pain and negative ultrasound (US) for acute cholecystitis.

BACKGROUND
Acute cholecystitis is the most common cause of acute right upper quadrant pain in patients presenting to hospital emergency rooms.

TEST RATIONALE
Most of the patients presenting to the emergency room with acute right upper quadrant pain undergo US as the first diagnostic imaging test. A stone impacted in the cystic duct is diagnostic of acute cholecystitis but this finding is rare (<5%). Although thickening of the gallbladder wall and the sonographic Murphy's sign are nonspecific, a combination of these signs in the presence of gallstones has an accuracy of approximately 90% for the diagnosis of acute cholecystitis. Nevertheless, these signs are often not clearly present in combination and confirmatory tests are needed. Technetium-99m IDA (iminodiacetic acid) cholescintigraphy (HIDA scan) is the study of choice for definitive diagnosis of acute cholecystitis with an accuracy of >95%, defining the underlying pathophysiology of the obstruction of the cystic duct.

Nonfilling of the gallbladder by 60 minutes after the tracer injection is abnormal. However, some patients will have delayed gallbladder filling up to 4 hours without acute cholecystitis. This prolonged scanning time can be reduced to 30 minutes by IV morphine augmentation (0.04 mg/Kg body weight) with the total scanning time of 90 minutes (see Fig. 10-2). Morphine causes constriction of the sphincter of Oddi and produces a 10-fold increase in the resting common bile duct pressure and preferential redirection of bile to the gall bladder.

Fasting or nonfatty diet only for more than 24 hours may produce a false-positive scan, as sludge may fill the gallbladder. In these cases, the patient should be pretreated with cholecystokinin (CCK) to empty the gall bladder before the tracer injection.

A false-negative scan can occur in the case of acalculous cholecystitis. If a false-negative scan due to an acalculous cholecystitis is suspected, CCK should be injected. Poor gallbladder contraction is indicative of acalculous cholecystitis, although it cannot differentiate between the acute and the chronic form of this gallbladder pathology. In any case, a gallblad-

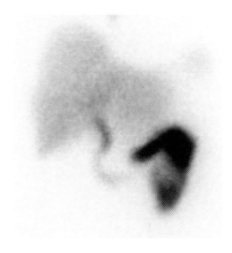

Figure 10-2 Nonvisualization of the gallbladder after 90 minutes (30 minutes after morphine augmentation), indicative of cystic duct obstruction.

der ejection fraction of less than 35% after CCK injection is predictive of symptomatic relief with cholecystectomy.

TEST OF CHOICE
Hepatobiliary (HIDA) scan.

BIBLIOGRAPHY
Harvey A. Zeisman, Janis P. O'Malley and James H. Thrall. *Nuclear Medicine, The Requisites*, 3rd edition. Philadelphia, PA: **Elsevier.** 2005:160-190.

10-3. Gastric Emptying

CASE HISTORY
A 64-year-old diabetic male presents with symptoms of bloating and nausea.

BACKGROUND
Certainty about the diagnosis of chronic functional delayed gastric emptying is important, considering considerable side effects of its treatment.

TEST RATIONALE
Chronic functional delayed gastric emptying is suspected in cases with mechanical obstruction such as a tumor, which is excluded by endoscopic and radiologic examinations, and in situations like long-standing diabetes mellitus and non ulcer related dyspepsia or as a side effect of drug therapy. Radionuclide gastric emptying study is a noninvasive method to measure the gastric emptying rate as a baseline and for follow-up after the start of a therapy (see Fig. 10-3). This test is easier to perform and more accurate than gastric dilutions methods or duodenal recovery methods. Accuracy of the test depends on the standardization of the methodology within the institution. This standardization includes definition of the test meal composition, meal volume, patient positioning (supine versus upright), frequency of data acquisition and study length, and also defines the normal gastric emptying values. Consensus recommendations have recently been published by national organizations, which are expected to improve interinstitutional comparison of the studies. Most nuclear medicine facilities use egg white labeled with Technetium-99m sulfur colloid as test meal. A liquid meal is reserved for patients who cannot tolerate solid food, including those in pediatric population. Knowledge of patient's medication at the time of the study is imperative in overall interpretation of the results. Overnight fasting is required for this study.

TEST OF CHOICE
Radionuclide gastric emptying study.

BIBLIOGRAPHY
Abell TL, Camilleri M, Donohoe K, et al. Consensus recommendations for gastric emptying scintigraphy: a joint report of the American Neurogastroenterology and Motility Society and the Society of Nuclear Medicine. *Am J Gastroenterol.* 2008;103(3):753-763.

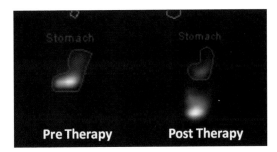

Figure 10-3   Anterior view of the stomach—delayed gastric emptying with calculated emptying of 11% at 120 minutes pretherapy and 100% at 120 minutes posttherapy with metoclopramide.

10-4. Thyroid Nodule

CASE HISTORY
A 23-year-old male presents with solitary thyroid nodule and indeterminate cytology result after fine needle aspiration.

BACKGROUND
Functional status of thyroid nodules (hyperfunctioning versus hypofunctioning or non functioning) helps to estimate of likelihood of malignancy in nodules with indeterminate cytology.

TEST RATIONALE
Less than 10% of all palpable thyroid nodules are malignant. The risk of malignancy increases in young people, in people older than 60 and in males and with growth of the nodule and after radiation to the neck and mediastinum. Fine needle aspiration (preferably with US guidance) is often the first diagnostic step. However, even in skilled hands and with an experienced cytopathologist, approximately 10% of aspirates are nondiagnostic. In such cases, a radionuclide thyroid scan is the next diagnostic step. A hyperfunctioning (or "hot") nodule is extremely unlikely (1%) to be malignant but a hypofunctioning (or "cold") nodule has a 10%–20% likelihood of being malignant and should undergo rebiopsy or surgical excision (see Fig. 10-4). A warm nodule; a nodule with the same level of uptake as the surrounding thyroid tissue is less likely to be malignant. But such a nodule may also represent a cold nodule located in the posterior aspect of the gland, appearing with normal level of uptake on the scan. A warm nodule may also need further evaluation, depending on the clinical presentation, size, and US findings. This scenario also underlines the importance of correlation between the findings on radionuclide thyroid scan and thyroid US.

A radionuclide thyroid scan is frequently performed with Technetium-99m pertechnetate and not with radioiodine. Compared with radioiodine, pertechnetate has the advantage of favorable radiation dosimetry and shorter study time (30 minutes versus up to 24 hours) but can delay the diagnosis, should a so-called discordant nodule (hot on pertechnetate scan and cold on radioiodine scan) be suspected. Pertechnetate is trapped in the thyroid but not organified and because some thyroid cancers are capable of trapping but lose the organification function, a single hot nodule on pertechnetate scan can represent a dilemma in certain circumstances, such as in pediatric population and young adults. Radioiodine is trapped and organified and should be used in cases of suspected discordant nodule for

Figure 10-4
Technetium-99m
pertechnetate thyroid scan
revealed a cold nodule
in the right lower pole
(arrow head). The patient
subsequently underwent
repeat ultrasound-guided
biopsy of the correspond-
ing isoechoic nodule.
The differential diagnosis
of the cytologic findings
included papillary carci-
noma. The final pathology
after total thyroidectomy
confirmed the diagnosis
of papillary thyroid carcinoma. The 123-I uptake
at 24 hours was 22.4%
(normal 15%–35%).

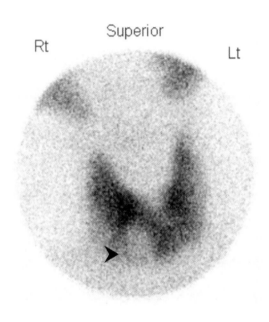

Superior

Rt

Lt

further assessment. A discordant nodule may also represent a benign lesion, such as follicular adenoma/adenomatous hyperplasia.

Thyroid scan is frequently combined with thyroid uptake measurement, especially in cases with low or suppressed thyroid stimulating hormone (TSH), since in such cases the severity of hyperfunction could determine the need for radioiodine therapy.

TEST OF CHOICE
Thyroid scan +/– thyroid uptake.

BIBLIOGRAPHY
Harvey A. Zeisman, Janis P. O'Malley and James H. Thrall. *Nuclear Medicine, The Requisites*, 3rd edition. Philadelphia, PA: Elsevier. 2005:88-92.
Taylor A, Schuster DM, Alazraki N. A clinician's guide to nuclear medicine. Society of Nuclear Medicine. 2000:181-198.
Wilson MA. *Text Book of Nuclear Medicine*. Philadelphia, PA: Lippincott-Raven. 1998:171-175.

10-5. Osteomyelitis

CASE HISTORY
A 57-year-old female diabetic presents with ulcer at the right heel and normal radiographs.

BACKGROUND
Osteomyelitis has to be confirmed (or excluded) with certainty before start of therapy.

TEST RATIONALE
Plain radiographs should be performed first when osteomyelitis is suspected. However, radiographic changes caused by osteomyelitis may take 14 days or even longer to develop. Bone scan is typically positive within 24 hours of the onset of osteomyelitis with a sensitivity of 95% so that a negative bone scan at this time practically excludes osteomyelitis (see Fig. 10-5). The specificity of bone scan is reduced in cases with underlying bone conditions, such as previous fracture or neuropathic joint. Bone scan can be combined with a radio labeled white blood scan to increase specificity. Gadolinium-enhanced MRI has similar sensitivity as bone scan but also the same limitations in regard to specificity. MRI has the advantage of better anatomic localization but is of limited use due to side effects associated with gadolinium administration, especially in patients with renal impairment, and also cannot be used in patients with metallic hardware. Bone scan has the additional advantage of whole-body survey, which is particularly useful in pediatric patients and in patients with fever of unknown origin. For better anatomic localization, bone scan can be performed as SPECT-CT (fused tomographic imaging of nuclear scan and CT).

TEST OF CHOICE
Three-phase bone scan (+/- SPECT-CT).

BIBLIOGRAPHY
Chew FS. *Musculoskeletal Imaging, the Core Curriculum.* Lippincott Williams & Wilkins, 2003:487-494.
Zeisman HA, O'Malley JP, Thrall JH. *Nuclear Medicine, the Requisites.* 3rd ed. Elsevier, 2005:404-407.

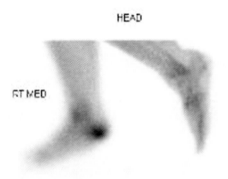

Figure 10-5 Uptake in the calcaneus on the delayed images, compatible with osteomyelitis.

10-6. Brain Lymphoma

CASE HISTORY
A 39-year-old male with acquired immunodeficiency syndrome (AIDS) presented with seizure and noted to have multiple brain lesions on CT.

BACKGROUND
Differentiating lymphoma from toxoplasmosis in patients with AIDS and brain lesions is necessary for proper therapy.

TEST RATIONALE
Lymphoma and toxoplasmosis are the two main differential diagnoses in AIDS patients presenting with brain lesions. These lesions are usually detected first on CT or MRI. Nevertheless, CT or MRI can often not reliably differentiate between lymphoma and toxoplasmosis, as both present as ring-enhancing lesions. Brain biopsy is the gold standard but often avoided due to associated morbidity and sampling error. 201-Thallium brain scan (with SPECT or SPECT-CT for tomographic imaging) is a noninvasive test with very high sensitivity (>95%) and specificity (>90%) that can reliably differentiate between these two entities. Lymphoma has intense Thallium uptake while toxoplasmosis does not (see Fig. 10-6). Thallium brain scan may not be reliable in lesions smaller than 2 cm (false-negative result). In such cases, FDG PET can be used to differentiate these two entities (lymphoma: intense FDG uptake; toxoplasmosis: low to absent uptake). Both Thallium and FDG are injected intravenously and images are acquired 10 and 60 minutes after injection, respectively. There is no preparation needed for Thallium scan whereas the patient must fast for 4 hours for FDG PET. In both scans, a false-positive result may occur with abscess, while partially treated and necrotic tumors and small size may cause false-negative result. Both Thallium scan and FDG PET should be obtained on hybrid scanners such as as SPECT-CT or PET-CT. This facilitates anatomic localization and the fused images can be directly used for radiation therapy planning.

TEST OF CHOICE
Thallium SPECT-CT (or FDG PET-CT).

BIBLIOGRAPHY
Andrew Taylor, David M. Schuster and Naomi Alazraki. A Clinician's Guide to Nuclear Medicine. Society of Nuclear Medicine. 2000:139-180.

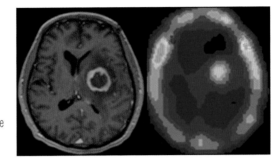

Figure 10-6 Ring-enhancing lesion in the region of the left basal ganglia indeterminate for lymphoma versus toxoplasmosis on MRI. Intense uptake on Thallium scan indicative of lymphoma.

10-7. Gastrointestinal Tract (GI) Bleed

CASE HISTORY
A 57-year-old male presents with bleeding per rectum.

BACKGROUND
Localization of the source of an acute lower GI bleed is necessary for proper therapy.

TEST RATIONALE
The source of a lower GI bleed is usually determined by endoscopy. However, lower GI bleed is frequently intermittent and as such difficult to localize by endoscopy. In such cases, a radionuclide bleeding scan, performed during the time of rectal bleed, has a high likelihood to localize the source of the bleed to the small bowel, cecum, ascending colon, hepatic flexure, transverse colon, splenic flexure, descending colon or rectosigmoid, and point the interventional radiologist toward the vessel involved for diagnostic and therapeutic purposes (see Fig. 10-7). Before ordering this test, an upper GI source of the rectal bleed should be excluded. In radionuclide bleeding scan, autologous red blood cell (RBC) is labeled with Technetium-99m and reinjected into the patient. Images are then acquired for 90 minutes to document extravasation of radiotracer into the bowel in case of active bleeding. The study is stopped when a bleeding source is visualized and the patient is rushed from nuclear medicine to interventional radiology for angiography. On the other hand, if no source of bleeding is seen within 90 minutes, the study can be repeated without reinjection within up to 24 hours. There is no special preparation needed for this study. The labeling process takes approximately 30 minutes, using a standard commercial kit, available in nuclear medicine departments.

TEST OF CHOICE
Radionuclide bleeding study.

BIBLIOGRAPHY
Harvey A. Zeisman, Janis P. O'Malley, James H. Thrall. *Nuclear Medicine, The Requisites*, 3rd edition. Elsevier, 2005:364-372.

Rt   Lt

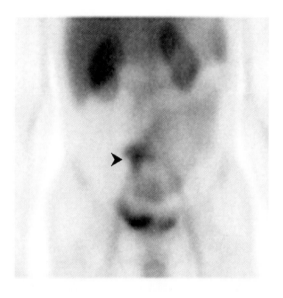

Figure 10-7   Uptake in
the small bowel (arrow
head) indicating the
location of the bleed.

10-8. Renal Obstruction

CASE HISTORY
A 56-year-old female presents with right-sided hydronephrosis after pelvic surgery.

BACKGROUND
Obstructive hydronephrosis should be promptly identified for early correction.

TEST RATIONALE
US is usually used to document hydronephrosis but cannot assess its urodynamic relevance. Diuretic renal scan is a noninvasive method to distinguish obstructive from nonobstructive hydronephrosis. In a dilated but not obstructed renal collecting system, increased urine flow after diuretic administration causes washout of radiotracer whereas obstruction prevents augmented washout. Diuretic renal scan can also be used to assess for obstruction before hydronephrosis has been manifested (immediately after surgery) or to assess for urodynamic relevance of hydroureter. Furthermore, diuretic renal scan can also be used to assess the effectiveness of the corrective measures such as stenting or surgery as well the relative function of each kidney (see Fig. 10-8). The latter is used in prenatal hydronephrosis as a parameter to determine the need for intervention when the function of the hydronephrotic kidney deteriorates.

In preparation for the study, the patient needs to be properly hydrated (500 ml orally, 30–60 minutes before radiotracer injection in adults) and void just before the start. Infants, children who cannot void voluntarily and adults with neurogenic bladder or bladder outlet obstruction need bladder catheterization, as retrograde flow could cause a false-positive result. A false-positive result can also be caused by vesicoureteral reflux. Other causes of a false-positive result include an extremely dilated collecting system and impaired renal function on the hydronephrotic side; delayed images after ambulation of the patient should be considered in the former case, and additional injection of diuretic prior to start of the scan (F-15 protocol) in the latter, although the study might be nondiagnostic in case of extremely poor renal function.

Furosemide (40 mg in adults; 1 mg/kg in infants and children, maximum 40 mg) is the diuretic of choice, injected intravenously over 1–2 minutes at 20 minutes after the start of the study (F+20 protocol) with the entire study lasting 40 minutes. However, protocols with injection of furosemide 15 minutes before (F-15 protocol) or together with the radiotracer (F+0 protocol) injection are in use. False-positive results in infants due to immaturity of kidneys and limited response to furosemide have been described.

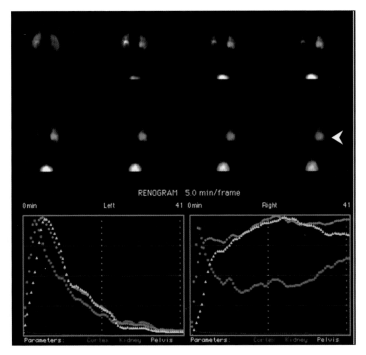

Figure 10-8   Intense and symmetric (right, 49%; left, 51%) uptake of radiotracer in both cortices indicating proper function bilaterally. There is also proper excretion on the left; whereas, the right side shows increasing accumulation of radiotracer in the renal pelvis with no improvement after furosemide (arrow head and yellow curve), indicating obstruction on the right.

Technetium-99m MAG3 (99m-Tc MAG3) is the tracer of choice due to superior image quality compared to Technetium-99m DTPA (99m-Tc DTPA), particularly in patients with diminished renal function.

TEST OF CHOICE
Diuretic renal scan.

BIBLIOGRAPHY
Harvey A. Zeisman, Janis P. O'Malley, James H. Thrall. *Nuclear Medicine, The Requisites*, 3rd edition. Elsevier, 2005:237-239.
Michael A. Wilson. *Text Book of Nuclear Medicine*. Lippincott-Raven. 1998:125-129.

10-9. Thyroid Disease

CASE HISTORY
A 20-year-old female presents with weight loss, palpitations, and suppressed TSH.

BACKGROUND
Grave's disease and subacute thyroiditis can often not be differentiated as etiology of newly diagnosed thyrotoxicosis.

TEST RATIONALE
Thyrotoxicosis is characterized by various combinations of weight loss, frequent bowel movements, heat intolerance, nervousness, sleeplessness, palpitations, hyperhidrosis and anxiety, and suppressed TSH. Despite clinical history (recent upper respiratory infection in thyroiditis) and physical examination (exophthalmus in Grave's disease and tender thyroid in thyroiditis) the underlying etiology often remains unclear. And since the managements for these conditions are completely different, thyroid uptake measurement is often needed to promptly make the correct diagnosis and initiate treatment.

High thyroid uptake (>50%) is indicative of Grave's disease and low uptake (<5%) is indicative of subacute thyroiditis (see Fig. 10-9). The test is preferably performed with radioiodine than with Technetium-99m pertechnetate, although the latter has the advantage of favorable radiation dosimetry (children) and shorter study time (30 minutes versus up to 24 hours). Radioiodine has the advantage of well-defined normal range (generally 10%–35% in the United States but may vary, depending on the local iodine supply in drinking water), which increases the diagnostic certainty and can also be used to calculate the radioiodine therapy dose, if therapy indicated for Grave's disease. Preference should also be given to 123-I over 131-I, again due to favorable radiation dosimetry. A patient needs to be fasting for 4 hours if radioiodine is given orally. Pertechnetate is given only by the intravenous route. Thyroid uptake is often combined with thyroid scan. The latter has the advantage of increasing the diagnostic certainty, although it is not absolutely necessary while differentiation Grave's disease from subacute thyroiditis. Some institutions use a very low dose of 131-I (lower cost than 123-I) for uptake measurement in combination with pertechnetate for the thyroid scan.

Thyroid uptake could be underestimated due to recent exposure to stable, nonradioactive iodine (iodinated contrast media or foods supplements). However, the decision as to perform the thyroid uptake measurement

RT

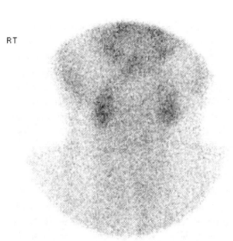

Figure 10-9 Thyroid uptake of 0.3% at 4 hours and 0.4% at 24 hours indicative of subacute thyroiditis. No tracer accumulation is seen in the thyroid bed region on the thyroid scan, further confirming the diagnosis of subacute thyroiditis.

should be based on the clinical necessity of the test, and the test should not be denied solely based on a history of exposure to stable iodine because the effect of such exposure on thyroid uptake is variable and often insignificant due to high iodine supply in drinking water in the United States.

TEST OF CHOICE
Thyroid uptake +/– thyroid scan.

BIBLIOGRAPHY
Harvey A. Zeisman, Janis P. O'Malley and James H. Thrall. *Nuclear Medicine, The Requisites*, 3rd edition. Elsevier, 2005:77-87.
Michael A. Wilson. *Text Book of Nuclear Medicine*. Lippincott-Raven. 1998:156-159.

INDEX

Page numbers in *italics* refer to figures and tables.